Ambulatory
Care

University Health Policy Consortium Series

In 1977, Boston University, Brandeis University, and the Massachusetts Institute of Technology established the University Health Policy Consortium to conduct health policy analyses and research projects and to provide an educational laboratory for students interested in health policy. A year later, the Health Care Financing Administration designated the Consortium as its first Center for Health Policy Analysis and Research. The Center concentrates its research in three major health-care areas: long-term care, health-care quality and effectiveness, and regulation and reimbursement.

Brandeis University is the host institution for the Consortium, which is housed at the Florence Heller Graduate School for Advanced Studies in Social Welfare. Both the Center and the Consortium bring together social scientists, lawyers, and medical personnel to conduct collaborative research in health care.

This book represents analyses that have been done by Consortium associates and other health-care professionals outside the Consortium community.

Other books in the UHPC series are:

Federal Health Programs
Edited by Stuart Altman and Harvey M. Sapolsky

Reforming the Long-Term-Care System
Edited by James J. Callahan, Jr., and Stanley S. Wallack

Rural Medicine
Stanley S. Wallack and Sandra E. Kretz

Regional Variations in Hospital Use
Edited by David L. Rothberg

Ambulatory Care

Problems of Cost and Access

Edited by
Stuart H. Altman
Joanna Lion
Judith LaVor Williams
University Health Policy
Consortium

LexingtonBooks
D.C. Heath and Company
Lexington, Massachusetts
Toronto

Library of Congress Cataloging in Publication Data
Main entry under title:

Ambulatory care.

(University Health Policy Consortium series)
Includes index.
1. Ambulatory medical care—United States. 2. Ambulatory medical
care—United States—Costs. I. Altman, Stuart H. II. Lion, Joanna.
III. Williams, Judith LaVor. IV. Series. [DNLM: 1. Ambulatory care—
Economics—United States. 2. Health policy—United States. WX 205 A497]
RA395.A3A495   1983   338.4′33621   82-49054
ISBN 0-669-06401-7

Published simultaneously in Canada

Printed in the United States of America

International Standard Book Number: 0-669-06401-7

Library of Congress Catalog Card Number: 82-49054

Contents

Tables

Acknowledgments

Ambulatory care has been a frequently overlooked element in the nation's rapidly growing investment in health care. The Robert Wood Johnson Foundation has, over the past decade, committed significant resources to the organization and study of ambulatory care. We are indebted to the foundation for its support of our research on the costs of ambulatory care at the Heller School over the past four years.

1

Policy Setting for
Ambulatory Care

Stuart H. Altman

U.S. hospitals and the groups responsible for health-care payment are approaching an impasse over the issue of whether ambulatory-care programs that are hospital based should be expanded or curtailed in the next decade. The impasse results from the seeming paradox that, on the one hand, hospital-sponsored ambulatory care is the fastest-growing component of hospital services while, on the other, such a delivery system represents the most expensive way of providing ambulatory care. While hospital planners are looking to ambulatory care as the major growth area for the 1980s, their counterparts in government are seeking, in the name of cost containment, ways of slowing or halting this growth.

The growth in ambulatory care is evidenced by significant expenditure increases over the past decade. Total personal-care expenditures rose from $60.8 billion in 1970 to $210.3 billion in 1980. In chapter 4, Schieber breaks down these expenditures: Physician visits rose from $13.5 billion to $45.0 billion in the same period, while hospital-outpatient care jumped from $1.7 billion to $9.9 billion, nearly a fivefold increase. The total number of OPD visits increased by 62 percent during this period.

Clearly, factors other than volume are at work here, some of which will be discussed further in this book. It should also be noted that *all* health-care expenditures rose during this period, so that the relative proportion comprising ambulatory care remained pretty much the same.

Medicare and Medicaid, according to Schieber, accounted for 30 percent of all hospital OPD reimbursements and for 21 percent of all physician-service payments in 1980. These figures have given rise to concern within the federal government and in such state governments as New York that the large and growing amounts they pay for hospital OPD care may be excessive and need to be curtailed. Not all third-party payers favor cutting back this form of care, however; private insurors such as Blue Cross and Blue Shield view it as a far less expensive substitute for a substantial amount of inpatient care. Hospitals argue that they provide needed, and sometimes the sole, ambulatory services for many groups, particularly the poor and minorities who live in inner cities. They point out the burden placed on them of treating a more difficult caseload, maintaining modern and high-quality facilities, and caring for a large number of nonpaying patients.

Issues of equity, access, and cost abound in the ambulatory-care field.

1

Although payment is really only part of the program, reimbursement looms large given the degree to which it can influence the growth and kinds of services provided and the importance of government involvement in the payment for ambulatory care. Problems are exacerbated by inconsistencies in reimbursement methods. Whereas Medicare pays physicians on a tightly constrained fee basis, hospital OPD services are paid on a charge basis with no arbitrary limits. Hence a shift in the focus of service could lead to sizeable increases in governmental expenditures.

In 1977 Congress considered legislation to limit Medicare payments to OPDs by pegging them to some multiple of average physician fees in the locale. Indeed, some states such as New York have set limits on Medicaid payments for hospital-based ambulatory care. These levels are considered by hospitals to be below the actual cost of the care. In fact, some have attributed the severe financial problems of a few New York City hospitals to the low rates of reimbursement for their ambulatory-care services.

In this environment of increasing costs and use of ambulatory care, and uncertainty over what to do about it, the Robert Wood Johnson Foundation asked the Heller School to undertake a review of what is known about ambulatory care costs, particularly how they compared in different settings. The Foundation had for years supported demonstration projects to strengthen the organization and delivery of ambulatory care by hospitals and saw a need to develop a better overall picture of the field. They had some concerns about the long-term viability of the hospital-related practices they were fostering, particularly when Foundation support elapsed and if reimbursement ceilings became fact. Based on some of the findings presented in this volume, these concerns may be justified.

The Foundation asked the Heller School to look into the following reasons why costs are alleged to vary across settings and to determine if such differences exist and their magnitude.

Overhead.   What percent of total OPD cost per visit can be attributed to costs allocated from inpatient departments?

Noncounterpart costs.   How do costs for areas of the hospital not used by outpatients affect overhead?

Research and education.   How do these factors affect costs?

Stand-by costs.   How much of a factor is additional personnel and staffing?

Medical case mix.   Are OPD patients actually physically sicker so that they require more physician time and other resources?

Psychosocial case mix.   Does the accepted fact that OPD patients have more problems than those in private practice necessarily mean that they use more resources?

It was the Foundation's hope that after a relatively brief period of research and literature review, a national commission could be established to develop definitive guidelines for reimbursement for ambulatory care. Further, there was hope that the Federal government would be willing to undertake a major, primary data-collection effort to fill knowledge gaps identified by the Heller project.

However, events in Washington precluded the data-collection effort, and the project's review indicated that there were substantial deficiencies in our knowledge, which rendered a national-policy commission infeasible at the time. There simply would not be enough facts available to reach sound conclusions about reimbursement policies.

The Heller School study was redirected toward filling some of the major information gaps, largely through analysis of existing data sources. Thus through most of the four-year project, we have been trying to shed light on the role in ambulatory-care costs of hospital-allocation procedures, elements of the cross-site cost differentials, and the case-mix issue.

As part of our plan for expanding our knowledge of both the costs and the delivery of various types of ambulatory care, as well as to share the findings from our own research, we decided to convene a conference. Our goal was to invite a small group of experts in the fields of ambulatory-care financing, policy, administration, and research in order to learn what others are doing and finding out and to obtain critiques of our work. Most of those we invited were able to attend the conference, which was held in June 1982.

The significance of the papers presented at the conference, as well as the discussions surrounding them, made the papers worthy of publication as a collection. A number of penetrating policy analyses and new findings from a number of research projects were presented for the first time.

Reimbursement Issues

The policy issues of the greatest significance revolved around reimbursement for ambulatory care and the need for reforms. Insurance coverage was one subject raised in this context. Davis cited the success of initiatives such as Medicare and Medicaid in improving access to care for the poor and aged, which ultimately raised health status. However, she pointed out, significant gaps in coverage remain, particularly for the poor and minorities. She views this as the most significant health-policy issue in the ambulatory-care field. Her findings were supported by representatives of the commercial insurance industry and Blue Cross/Blue Shield who believe we should be increasing coverage of ambulatory care and preventive services as a way to save on inpatient services.

The federal and state officials present at the conference zeroed in on reimbursement problems that have often created adverse incentives and led to piecemeal, and at times contradictory, reforms. Schieber points out that Medicare-reimbursement policies make outpatient-care costs difficult to control. While there are limits on inpatient routine costs, the OPD is not subject to those limits, being paid instead through a system based on charges. Furthermore, physicians are reimbursed on a fee-for-service basis even in the OPD and have few incentives to control ancillary procedures that generate increased revenues for them and the hospital.

Young seconds this problem by reviewing changing technologies and medical practices, which in turn often change the care setting. Although Medicare and Medicaid have made some adjustments in terms of coverage of what were formerly inpatient procedures, reimbursement practices have not been similarly reexamined. For example, the fees paid to physicians in private practice do not necessarily take into account the new technologies and increasingly sophisticated equipment found in physician's offices. Problems to be solved include how to determine payment levels, what equipment should be covered, and how to prevent duplicate billing when services are provided by more than one individual or group.

Although the need to drastically reform the ways in which ambulatory care is reimbursed, the path to doing so is not clear. The federal government has stated its intent to set limits on outpatient reimbursements, and one promising method is to devise ambulatory-visit groupings similar to the Diagnostic Related Groupings (DRGs) recently enacted as the method for paying for inpatient services.

From a state perspective, Crane and Salsberg cite some of the problems resulting from rate setting based on flat-fee schedules. Low physician fees and payment of OPDs on the basis of a prospectively determined, all-inclusive flat rate has reduced the number of private physicians willing to care for Medicaid recipients and created serious financial problems for some hospitals. Large numbers of medically indigent, who become bad debts in OPDs, exacerbate the problems. Congressman Rangel and Birns elaborate on these issues as they affect inner-city hospitals and access to health care by inner-city inhabitants.

Organizational Aspects

The past decade has seen substantial activity in the organization, and reorganization, of ambulatory care. Not only are more physicians joining together to practice in groups, but these groups are becoming larger, and many have developed into health-maintenance organizations (HMOs) with pre-paid capitation for their patients. One of the most significant organizational changes, however, has been the hospital OPD. Hospitals are not only expanding their activities but are moving away from the clinic image to try to build a sophisticated, attractive, and cost-efficient primary-care OPD. The Robert Wood Johnson Foundation has supported many of these activities through its demonstrations to foster primary-care group practices in community hospitals, teaching hospitals, and free-standing clinics related to minicipal hospitals.

Burns set the stage for this section of the conference by discussing trends in the organization of hospital outpatient care, describing such forms as hospital-operated facilities, contracted services, and the hospital as land-lord. Clearly, hospitals are increasingly seeing the OPD as a way to generate additional revenues; and given the different reimbursement policies just discussed, it may also be possible to shift costs to the OPD. One of the early prototypes of a primary-care group practice was Boston's Beth Israel Hospital. Winsten, Makadon, and Delbanco make some valuable points in chapter 9 about an innovative primary-care OPD, including the role of the OPD in generating ancillary-service revenue and in filling inpatient beds in a low-occupancy situation, both attributes that could enhance its value to the hospital. Sophisticated management techniques have been instituted and a stable patient load developed. On the other hand, other researchers suggest that the location of the OPD within the hospital leads to inefficiencies for the OPD when service, teaching, and research requirements come into the picture, and to higher costs if the hospital were to add in overhead based on standard cost-allocation techniques.

Several of the chapters in this book present valuable new findings on the progress of new organizational arrangements for hospital OPDs, but they also give cause for concern. How viable financially will all these hospital-affiliated, primary-care group practices be when seed money runs out? Two analyses of RWJF demonstration programs give some evidence that many of these OPD arrangements may not be able to make it on their own or else will need significantly more start-up time to become financially independent.

Wickizer and Shortell report their preliminary findings for the community hospital group-practice demonstrations. It does not appear that the new arrangements have significantly reduced nonurgent use of emergency rooms in the same hospitals, nor have the practices appeared to have much of an impact on the sponsoring hospital such as increasing use of its ancillary services. Financial-viability figures were not very encouraging either. The most striking finding is that, while the average number of visits per full-time equivalent physician doubled over the four-year period, this increase in efficiency and resulting drop in direct cost were not enough. After four years in operation, none of the practices was breaking even.

Wickizer and Shortell report that the average cost per visit dropped from over $72 in the first year to about $31 in the third year for the eleven hospitals in the preliminary analysis. These, it should be noted, are direct costs only; we do not know what the picture would be if indirect costs were added in. The same is true for Winsten, Makadon, and Delbanco, who report Beth Israel's OPD direct costs, including physician time, as being about $44 a visit with net revenue per visit being $44.49. These amounts are in line with the new findings of Henderson and Hannon who found a mean of $21.73 direct cost per visit, *exclusive* of physician costs, in 106 California general hospitals with OPDs.

Brecher et al. report similar results of slow development, problems in building caseload and high costs resulting from these, plus high construction and equipment costs. The fifteen free-standing, municipal hospital-sponsored clinics they looked at were established to try to draw patients out of costly emergency rooms and hospital OPDs. Findings on use of the clinic revealed a small proportion of the target area using these facilities compared with private practices and considerably less patient satisfaction with the public clinics.

Organizational and political problems with the local governments appeared to contribute to problems and delays. The question then is: What does it take to make the OPD fiscally viable while providing quality care?

A further question not addressed by these studies is the impact on total OPD costs of indirect costs since they have been factored out of the analyses. For example, the actual overhead rate that would apply to the OPD, discussed by Winsten, Makadon, and Delbanco, is not available, but the OPD and hospital have negotiated a rate equivalent to 30 percent of total costs. With this factored in and amounting to $18.42, the total Beth Israel Ambulatory Care cost per visit becomes $62.42, exclusive of tests, and the expected reimbursement per visit $44.49. This reimbursement includes indirect costs. A similar caveat applies to the OPDs studied by Wickizer and Shortell. Thus OPDs are more expensive overall than is indicated by their quoted direct costs.

Henderson and Hannon did calculate the overhead as well as the direct costs, coming up with $36.92 for all costs combined for all California hospitals. For the largest, which were primarily teaching hospitals in California, and are the most comparable to the hospital described by Winsten, Makadon, and Delbanco, the figure was $49.41; this was virtually identical with what Winsten, Makadon, and Delbanco found.

Getting a Fix on Cost Elements

The original mission of the Heller School project on the costs of ambulatory care was to identify the nature and extent of cost differences between hospital OPDs and private physicians' offices. This has proved much more difficult than we anticipated not only because of the lack of solid data but also because of different methods of defining and allocating costs. Nevertheless, some information has recently come to light through analyses of existing data as well as a small original data-collection effort.

Henderson and Hannon compare the elements making up the cost of a visit in hospital OPDs with those involved in primarily fee-for-service, medium-sized and large group practices. The average nonphysician cost per visit in the hospital was found to be significantly higher than the group practices' per-visit cost. However, contrary to some expectations, most of the differences were attributable to higher salary costs in the OPD. The larger the hospital, the higher the salary costs. Very little of the across-site cost differential was found to be due to plant and supplies, while a small part of the differential was due to costs peculiar to the hospital setting. This finding flies in the face of some of the conventional wisdom about what factors account for the cost differential.

Case-mix differences are frequently cited as one of the major factors in the cost differential. We are fortunate to have in this book two analyses of the role actually played by case mix. Lion and Williams review past research on ambulatory case mix, looking first at medical case-mix findings from an analysis of a large-scale national survey. They then report findings from a recently completed data collection in three teaching-hospital OPDs. Diagnoses are compared between the national study and the local one, which was adapted from the former.

The medical case-mix analysis from the national study reveals extremely small differences between OPDs and private practices, with OPD patients only slightly sicker. Although socioeconomic data are not available for private-practice patients, the authors examined the differential use of provider time within the OPD, by those with and without social problems. When diagnosis is held constant, patients with social problems use about 25 percent more provider time than those without. Even taken together, however, medical and socioeconomic problems appear to account for well under half of all additional costs in the OPD.

The original findings of this study, when first published, created considerable controversy, especially among the medical directors of large teaching hospitals, and occasioned some discussion at the conference. It was partially in response to this feeling that the initial findings were not representative of teaching hospitals and their problems that the research reported on in chapter 13 was undertaken in three large teaching hospitals. The value of the conference was borne out in this way since the gut feeling of the teaching hospitals—that their patients were more complicated to treat—turned out to be true in the special study, although these complications appear to be attributed more to social than to medical problems.

Somewhat different findings, though not necessarily contradictory ones, came from a study by Held and Swartz. Using data for a Medicaid population in California of aid to families with dependent children (AFDC) recipients and disabled, they looked at hospitalization rates for patients whose primary source of ambulatory care was a hospital OPD or a private physician's office.

Overall analysis showed significantly higher hospitalization rates for OPD patients, indicating either a much sicker case mix or differences in medical practice across sites. However, when pregnancies and deliveries are omitted, the differences evaporate, indicating that OPD patients do not appear to be much sicker than private-practice patients. Held and Swartz argue, though, that the presence of a large number of pregnant women in the OPD caseload does mean that the case mix among settings is substantially different. The findings from the various data sources and analyses which Lion and Williams reported on are all limited to primary care visits.

Conclusion

The information in this book, and the issues raised in it, reinforce the fact that the problems of ambulatory care are the problems of health care and that solutions in the former are going to be inseparable from actions on overall health-policy issues. Some questions, however, seem unique to ambulatory care such as the appropriate social policy and equity.

What are the public's social expectations for health care? Should outpatient services be different depending on the patient's income and location? Or can we structure a uniform system of ambulatory care for all people? Should hospital OPDs cease to exist because of the fact that they indisputably cost more than other settings?

While hospital OPD costs *are* higher, there are many reasons for these differences, and they are not likely to disappear. For example, hospitals, unlike physicians' offices, are complex bureaucratic organizations that maintain large administrative staffs, teaching and research facilities, and so on. It is unreasonable to expect a hospital to turn out the same product at the same cost as the private physician. Other factors have already been described in this chapter.

If hospital-based ambulatory care is the only care available to many elderly, indigent, and minority patients, society must decide whether it wants to continue to provide this access to care for these groups. If we need and wish to maintain these kinds of services, we must be willing to pay for more expensive care. One question yet to be answered, though, is how much more expensive does it really need to be, or how much more is society, through government, willing to pay?

Other problems raised at the conference include some "backsliding" in terms of coverage and reimbursement for services, largely as a result of budget constraints. Fears were expressed that these cutbacks would create problems of access or lead back to a two-class system of care. While some conferees were concerned about impending hospital closings, others said they would survive by increasing competition for "the paying patients." Access to care, and types of services offered, could be reduced as a result of rate-setting efforts that limit reimbursements.

Divergent trends and interests were cited in ambulatory care in particular, as well as health care in general. The various aims involved, it was predicted, will set very different agendas. Physicians will seek legislation to address the oversupply of doctors and to maintain their incomes. Private corporations as well as many physicians will want to slow down public programs and decrease their health-insurance costs.

Similarly, insurors will attempt to prevent cost shifting from patients who can not pay for their care to insurors who are obliged to pay. All these parties will be going to their legislators in the future to seek solutions that benefit them.

These are competing problems and interests and will demand solutions that may conflict. The purpose of bringing together the varied participants at this conference was to try to deal with the divergent interests, find out what is known and what is going on, and try to form overall solutions rather than more piecemeal measures that will lead to new problems.

The tentative conclusions reached after a review of all the findings in this book is that the problem of hospital OPD costs is not a single item. It is not simply overhead, nor is it medical or socioeconomic case mix. There are, to be sure, differences, but no single one appears to be significant. The chapters in this book also point out a substantial amount of activity in the reorganization of hospital OPDs in an attempt to create more fiscally viable organizations for ambulatory care. These include hospital-based group practices, free-standing clinics, HMOs, and so on.

Not all these innovations will survive, but the system is clearly responding to new stimuli and the pressures of an increasingly constrained supply of funds. This willingness to change has to be an encouraging development and one that should be fully understood by those responsible for developing a new ambulatory-care-reimbursement system.

Part I
Access to Care

2

Public-Policy Implications

Karen Davis

Major gains have been made in the last fifteen years in access to ambulatory care for many disadvantaged population groups: the poor, residents of rural areas, and members of minority racial and ethnic groups. This progress is in large part attributable to major federal health programs initiated in the mid-1960s, including Medicaid, Medicare, and community health centers, followed in the early 1970s by the enactment of the National Health Service Corps.

These programs, however, stop short of reaching everyone experiencing financial or physical barriers to access to care. Medicaid covers only 40 percent of those with incomes below the federal poverty level.[1] Community health centers and communities served by National Health Service Corps physicians and other health professionals reach only 6 million out of 20 million residents of high-poverty, medically underserved, rural and inner-city areas.[2]

For those falling outside the reach of current programs, major gaps in access to care remain. Lack of health-insurance coverage in low-income groups is a particularly serious problem. These groups frequently go without needed care or, in urban areas, rely on crowded public-hospital facilities for care in emergencies.

This chapter summarizes the progress that has been made in improving access to care for disadvantaged groups, presents new data on remaining gaps for special population groups, summarizes the experience of federal ambulatory-care programs, and concludes with recommendations for future public policy to ensure access to ambulatory care for all.

Access to Ambulatory Care: The Current Evidence

With the investment in primary care made by federal programs in the late 1960s and the 1970s, significant progress in improving access to primary care for the poor and other disadvantaged groups was achieved. Numerous studies have been conducted examining trends in access to health care. Virtually all studies conclude that differentials, by income, in use of physician services and preventive service have narrowed.[3] Some authors go further and conclude that the evidence indicates that all significant gaps have been eliminated and access to health care is universally shared. While this overstates the success of federal programs, it is clear that much has been achieved.

In the early 1960s the nonpoor visited physicians 23 percent more frequently than the poor, despite the fact that then, as now, the poor were considerably sicker than the nonpoor. By the late 1970s the poor visited physicians more frequently than the nonpoor, and they did so more in accordance with their greater need for health-care services. Blacks and other minorities also made substantial gains over this period. Use of services by rural residents also increased relative to urban residents.[4]

Use of preventive services by the poor, minorities, and rural residents continues to lag well behind those not facing similar barriers to health care. Some studies have also found that when adjusted for the greater health needs of the disadvantaged, differentials continue to exist for all disadvantaged groups.[5]

The major difficulty with past studies, however, is that they have not examined the cumulative effect of lack of financial and physical access to care. How do uninsured blacks in rural areas fare in obtaining ambulatory-care services? Is it the case that nearly all disadvantaged people can get care from public hospitals or clinics, or do those facing multiple barriers to care simply do without?

New data from the 1977 National Medical Care Expenditure Survey (NMCES) shed some light on the cumulative effect of multiple barriers to care. The NMCES survey is based on interviews with a nationwide sample of approximately 40,000 people. This survey finds that 22 to 25 million people are uninsured for some time during the year but also notes that, of those, 18 million are uninsured during the entire year and as many as 35 million are uninsured at least some time during the year.[6] The uninsured are predominantly low income. Minorities are less likely to be insured than are whites. Sixteen percent of Hispanics are uninsured, and 10 percent of blacks, compared to 7 percent of whites. Residents of rural areas are 50 percent more likely to be uninsured than are residents of metropolitan areas.

Insurance coverage does have a marked effect on use of ambulatory care. Table 2–1 presents data from NMCES for the population under age sixty-five (the elderly are excluded from this chapter since nearly all the elderly are covered by Medicare and have some minimal financial coverage for ambulatory care). As shown, the insured average 3.7 visits with physicians during the year, compared with 2.4 visits for the uninsured (the NMCES survey does not include telephone contacts in visit counts). That is, the insured receive 54 percent more ambulatory care from physicians than do the uninsured.

Residence and race further affect use of ambulatory services. The lowest use of ambulatory care occurs for blacks and other minorities (includ-

Table 2–1
Physician Visits per Person under Sixty-Five per Year, by Insurance Status, Residence, and Race, 1977

Residence and Race	Uninsured	Insured	Ratio
Total	2.4	3.7	1.54
South	2.1	3.5	1.67
White	2.3	3.7	1.61
Black and other	1.5	2.8	1.87
Nonsouth	2.6	3.8	1.46
White	2.7	3.8	1.41
Black and other	1.9	3.5	1.84
SMSA	2.4	3.8	1.58
White	2.6	3.9	1.50
Black and other	1.7	3.2	1.88
NonSMSA	2.3	3.3	1.43
White	2.4	3.4	1.42
Black and other	1.6	2.9	1.81

Source: Data from the U.S. Department of Health and Human Services, National Center for Health Services Research, National Medical Care Expenditure Survey.

ing Hispanics). For blacks and other minorities without insurance coverage, use of ambulatory services is less than one-half the level of care received by more advantaged groups. For example, uninsured blacks and other minorities in the South receive 1.5 physician visits per person annually, compared with 3.7 physician visits for insured whites in the South. That is, to be multiply advantaged leads to use rates almost 2.5 times that of those who are multiply disadvantaged.

Insurance coverage reduces much, but not all, of the differential use of ambulatory services. Insured blacks in the South, for example, average 2.8 physician visits annually, compared with 3.5 for whites in the South. That is, whites average about 25 percent more ambulatory care than blacks and other minorities even if both are insured.

Rural residents receive somewhat less care than urban residents, whether white or black. Among insured groups, rural whites receive 3.4 physician visits annually compared with 3.9 visits for urban whites. Rural blacks and other minorities receive 2.9 physician visits compared with 3.2 visits for their insured counterparts in urban areas.

Insurance is particularly helpful in improving access to care for minorities. Insured minorities receive 80 to 90 percent more ambulatory care than do uninsured minorities, both in rural areas and in urban areas.

Despite the common perception that all disadvantaged people can obtain hospital care from some charity facility, tremendous differentials in use of hospital care also exist by insurance status, residence, and race. As shown in table 2–2, the insured receive 90 percent more hospital care than do the uninsured. Differentials by insurance status are particularly marked in the South and in rural areas. In the South the insured receive three times as many days of hospital care annually as do the uninsured, regardless of race or ethnicity.

Lower use of ambulatory and inpatient care by the uninsured is not a reflection of lower need for health-care services. Instead, as measured by self-assessment of health status, the uninsured tend to be somewhat sicker than the insured. As shown in table 2–3, 15 percent of the uninsured rate their health as fair or poor, compared with 11 percent of the insured. Blacks and other minorities in the South systematically rate their health the worst. Of uninsured blacks and other minorities in the South, 19 percent assess their health as fair or poor, compared with 9 percent of insured whites out-side the South.

Use of ambulatory services adjusted for the greater health needs of the uninsured and minorities shows even greater differentials. As shown in table 2–4, physician visits per person under age sixty-five in fair or poor health average 6.9 among the insured, compared to 4.1 visits for the uninsured with similar health problems. Insured blacks and other minorities with fair or poor health receive twice as much care as uninsured blacks and other minorities with fair or poor health.

Table 2–2
Hospital Patient Days per 100 Persons under Sixty-Five, by Insurance Status, Residence, and Race, 1977

Residence and Race	Uninsured	Insured	Ratio
Total	47	90	1.91
South	35	104	2.97
White	33	100	3.03
Black and other	40	119	2.98
Nonsouth	56	84	1.50
White	51	81	1.59
Black and other	89	114	1.28
SMSA	50	86	1.72
White	44	83	1.89
Black and other	70	106	1.51
NonSMSA	42	99	2.36
White	43	94	2.19
Black and other	39	175	4.49

Source: Data from the U.S. Department of Health and Human Services, National Center for Health Services Research, National Medical Care Expenditure Survey.

Table 2–3
Percent of Persons under Sixty-Five with Fair or Poor Health,
by Insurance Status, Residence, and Race, 1977

Residence and Race	Uninsured (Percent)	Insured (Percent)	Ratio
Total	15	11	1.33
South	18	14	1.30
White	18	13	1.40
Black and other	19	19	1.00
Nonsouth	12	10	1.24
White	12	9	1.35
Black and other	12	17	.71
SMSA	13	11	1.21
White	12	10	1.29
Black and other	15	18	.88
NonSMSA	17	12	1.45
White	17	11	1.50
Black and other	17	18	.94

Source: Data from the U.S. Department of Health and Human Services, National Center for Health Services Research, National Medical Care Expenditure Survey.

Table 2–4
Physician Visits per Person under Sixty-Five in Fair or Poor Health
per Year, by Insurance Status, Residence, and Race, 1977

Residence and Race	Uninsured	Insured	Ratio
Total	4.1	6.9	1.68
South	3.8	6.1	1.61
White	4.4	6.4	1.45
Black and other	2.2	5.0	2.27
Nonsouth	4.5	7.4	1.64
White	4.6	7.6	1.65
Black and other	3.5	6.5	1.86
SMSA	4.1	7.2	1.76
White	4.7	7.6	1.62
Black and other	2.3	5.9	2.57
NonSMSA	4.2	6.3	1.50
White	4.3	6.4	1.49
Black and other	3.2	5.4	1.69

Source: Data from the U.S. Department of Health and Human Services, National Center for Health Services Research, National Medical Care Expenditure Survey.

The NMCES data confirm other studies that have found that disadvantaged groups are less likely to have a usual source of ambulatory care, are more likely to receive their care from a hospital OPD or a clinic than from a physician's office, and are more likely to travel longer and wait longer for care. For example, as illustrated in table 2–5, 84 percent of the insured have a physician's office as their usual source of care, compared with 67 percent of the uninsured. About 50 percent of uninsured blacks and other minorities have a physician's office as their usual source of care. While quite low in comparison to other groups, this does not fit the stereotype that all minorities in urban areas receive the bulk of their care from public facilities. Insurance coverage significantly increases the proportion of minorities who have a physician's office as their usual source of care. This finding would suggest that Medicaid coverage, for example, enables a substantial number of minorities to obtain care in a physician's office.

When they are able to obtain care, the uninsured must travel longer distances to obtain care than the insured. As shown in table 2–6, 25 percent of the uninsured travel 30 minutes or more to obtain care, compared to 18 percent of the insured. Differentials in travel time between the insured and uninsured are somewhat more marked in rural areas than in urban areas but are a problem for the uninsured everywhere. These data suggest that not only do the uninsured receive less care but when they do obtain care, they do

Table 2–5
Percent of Persons under Sixty-Five Whose Usual Source of Care Is a Physician's Office, by Insurance Status, Residence, and Race, 1977

Residence and Race	Uninsured (Percent)	Insured (Percent)	Ratio
Total	67	84	1.25
South	66	81	1.22
White	70	82	1.16
Black and other	53	76	1.41
Nonsouth	68	85	1.25
White	70	86	1.22
Black and other	45	69	1.53
SMSA	63	82	1.31
White	66	84	1.27
Black and other	49	71	1.43
NonSMSA	73	86	1.19
White	76	87	1.15
Black and other	52	79	1.53

Source: Data from the U.S. Department of Health and Human Services, National Center for Health Services Research, National Medical Care Expenditure Survey.

Table 2–6
Percent of Persons under Sixty-Five Traveling More than
Twenty-Nine Minutes to Receive Medical Care, by Insurance
Status, Residence, and Race, 1977

Residence and Race	Uninsured (Percent)	Insured (Percent)	Ratio
Total	25	18	1.39
South	29	21	1.39
White	30	20	1.48
Black and other	28	26	1.09
Nonsouth	21	16	1.29
White	22	16	1.35
Black and other	17	21	.81
SMSA	22	17	1.27
White	21	16	1.32
Black and other	24	24	1.00
NonSMSA	29	20	1.46
White	30	20	1.50
Black and other	23	19	1.24

Source: Data from the U.S. Department of Health and Human Services, National Center for Health Services Research, National Medical Care Expenditure Survey.

so by searching out over a longer distance for providers willing to see them.

In short, lack of insurance coverage is the major barrier to access to care. It affects markedly the amount of ambulatory and inpatient care received. Without insurance coverage, many individuals obviously do without care. For those able to obtain care, it means incurring substantial travel and waiting times.

The lack of insurance coverage has three major consequences: It contributes to unnecessary pain, suffering, disability and death among the uninsured; it places a financial burden on those who struggle to pay burdensome medical bills; and it places a financial strain on hospitals, physicians, and other health-care providers who attempt to provide care to the uninsured.

Research is limited on the current and long-term effects for the people who lack health-insurance coverage. This chapter gives extensive data on use patterns by the uninsured, disaggregated by residence and race; these data are being presented virtually for the first time. However, a number of recent studies have shown that medical-care use has a dramatic impact on health. A recent Urban Institute report by Hadley explores the relationship between medical-care use and mortality rates.[7] This study contains persuasive evidence that use of medical-care services leads to a marked reduction in mortality rates. A recent study by Goldman and Grossman at the

National Bureau of Economic Research has found that infant-mortality rates have dropped significantly in communities served by federally funded community health centers.[8] This growing body of evidence does provide considerable support to the importance of medical-care use in assuring a healthy population—and at least indirectly provides a basis for concern that the lower use of medical care by the uninsured contributes to unnecessary death and lowered health status.

Lack of insurance coverage also imposes serious financial burdens on those who try to make regular payments to retire enormous debts incurred in obtaining medical care. It also jeopardizes the financial stability of the limited number of hospitals and ambulatory-care providers willing to provide charity care for those unable to pay.

Alternative Ambulatory-Care Settings

Since the mid-1960s the federal government has supported programs to assist especially disadvantaged groups in obtaining access to health-care services.While the Medicaid program provides financing for ambulatory and inpatient services for a portion of the poor, it was recognized that minorities and residents face especially serious problems that could not be addressed simply by extending insurance coverage.

To improve access to care for these population groups, the federal government supported the development of primary care centers in rural and inner-city areas. Approximately 80 percent of those served by these centers are members of minority groups.[9] Centers are located in high-poverty areas and serve populations with multiple and complex health problems. In the 1970s this program was complemented by the National Health Service Corps program, which provides many of the physicians, dentists, and other health professionals that staff federally funded primary-care centers.

While direct-delivery programs for the underserved have been controversial, they have proven to be cost-effective approaches to providing high-quality ambulatory care to the poor.[10] Major savings in total cost of care for the population served are achieved in large part because patients cared for through the primary-care centers are hospitalized at a lower rate.

The cost effectiveness of this alternative form of ambulatory care has not been well understood. Early publicity about community health centers highlighted the high cost per visit to the centers. These criticisms compared the per-visit cost of a comprehensive range of services (including dental care, prescription drugs, transportation, and outreach) to a physician's fee for a routine visit. Despite the inappropriateness of the comparison, serious attempts were made to improve the efficiency of center operations. As a result, between 1974 and 1979, the health centers increased provider productivity by 32 percent, decreased administrative costs by 25 percent, decreased the cost per encounter by 25 percent, and increased reimbursements from third-party payers by 121 percent.[11]

The latest figures indicate that community-health-center costs for medical care including administrative cost per patient visit averaged $23 in FY 1980. Physician fees for an initial office visit are estimated to be $34 in 1980 and $21 for a follow-up office visit.[12] Thus, even on this basis, health-center costs would appear to compare favorably with private-physician charges.

Health-center costs including laboratory, x-ray, and pharmacy as well as medical and administrative costs averaged $36 per visit in 1980 ($39 per visit when transportation and other support services are included).[13] No comparable figures are available for patients receiving care from private physicians.

On an annual basis, health-center medical and administrative costs averaged $69 per person. This was compared with an expected annual expenditure per capita on physician's services of $198 for all U.S. residents in 1980.[14] Annual community-health-center costs per user for medical services, laboratory, x-ray, and pharmacy services averaged $108 in 1980, compared to $278 for this range of services for all U.S. residents. While it is difficult to make precise comparisons, it is clear that ambulatory care for community-health-center users costs considerably less than the same care for the population as a whole.

The major savings accruing to this form of ambulatory-care delivery, however, is the experience of health centers in lowering hospitalization rates of patients served by centers. Several earlier studies in various sites documented this lower hospitalization rate. One recent study by Freeman and Goetsch provides more systematic data on community-health-center users in comparison to other low-income groups.[15] The Freeman-Goetsch study is based on data for 1975 in five urban sites: Atlanta; Boston; Charleston (South Carolina); Kansas City; and East Palo Alto. This survey of 20,863 people obtained information on age, sex, race, education, income, insurance coverage, health status, primary source of care, and health-services use. Hospital-admission rates for those using community health centers as a primary source of care are 31 percent lower than for all those surveyed, and days of hospital care are 50 percent lower for community-health-center users than for the group as a whole. People who use hospital OPDs as a primary source of care are particularly high users of inpatient hospital services. Total days of care per capita for people using community health centers are about 70 percent lower than for those using hospital OPDs and almost 50 percent lower than for those obtaining care from private physicians.

Some of the differences in hospitalization may be attributable to other factors. For example, users of hospital OPDs may have more serious health conditions. A regression analysis of hospitalization rates holding constant for the effects of age, sex, race, education, income, insurance coverage, and health status (as measured by the presence or absence of a chronic condition), however, also reveals significantly lower hospitalization rates for community-health-center users. Holding constant for the preceding factors, hospital-admission rates are 50 percent lower for community-health-center users than for those who use hospital OPDs or emergency rooms as a primary source of care, and 30 percent lower than for those who use private physicians as a primary source of care. Those without any usual source of care have lower hospitalization rates, although this finding may reflect underutilization of health services.

Community-health-center patients use ambulatory-care services at the same rate as those obtaining care from hospital OPDs. People receiving care from private physicians have slightly higher use of ambulatory services, whereas patients with no usual source of care or those who rely on hospital emergency rooms have much lower rates of ambulatory-care use.

These results suggest that community health centers may be a lower-cost source of care, if cost is viewed as the total cost of all health services per person including hospitalization. Since inpatient hospitalization is one of the most costly components of care, the very substantial reduction in hospitalization for patients using community health centers as a source of care has important implications for public programs such as Medicaid.

The lower cost of community health centers does not appear to have been achieved through a deterioration of quality or underutilization of health-care services. Studies that have examined the quality of care have found health centers to provide high-quality care, surpassing most traditional settings for health care.[16] More recent studies have found that community health centers have contributed significantly to the reduction of infant mortality in the communities they serve.[17]

Policy Implications

Medicaid and primary-care centers have enabled many disadvantaged people to obtain ambulatory care. Yet many millions of people in need still fall outside these programs. For these people serious gaps persist in access to ambulatory care.

Recent policy measures are likely to exacerbate this situation.[18] The Omnibus Budget Reconciliation Act of 1981 reduced federal financial participation in Medicaid and curtailed eligibility under the AFDC program. Actions by state governments in response to this legislation could swell the ranks of the uninsured poor by over 1 million people. Coupled with the highest rate of unemployment since the Great Depression and the loss of health-insurance coverage frequently occurring with unemployment, the access problems of the uninsured are a pressing source of policy concern.

Simultaneously with the cutbacks in Medicaid, major reductions were made in community-health-center and migrant-health-center programs. Overall funding was reduced by 25 percent in absolute dollars, which may lead to a reduction of 1.1 million people served, out of a total population of 6 million served in 1980. The National Health Service Corps, although not as seriously affected at the present, will be substantially reduced in future years since no new scholarships are being awarded with commitments in underserved areas.

Financial strains on public hospitals and clinics supported by state and local governments are leading to further curtailment of services. Teaching hospitals that have for years maintained an opendoor policy are reevaluating the fiscal viability of continuing such a policy.

Recent hearings have documented the refusal of community hospitals to take uninsured patients, even in emergency situations.[19] This policy has led to documented cases of deaths that could have been avoided with prompt medical attention.

Such disparity in access to care is unacceptable in a decent and humane society. Several actions are required to assure progress toward adequate access to care for all. These include:

Expansion of Medicaid coverage to provide a coverage floor for all low-income people.

Continued funding and expansion of the community- and migrant-health-center programs to assure physical access to services for residents of high poverty, medically underserved communities.

Reform of Medicaid, Medicare, and private-health-insurance plans to encourage outpatient services in cost-effective, programs for primary care.

Experimentation with Medicaid capitation payments to primary-care centers, or networks of primary-care centers, to further encourage centers to reduce costly hospitalization.

Notes

1. United States Department Health and Human Services, Health Care Financing Administration, *Medicare and Medicaid Data Book, 1981*, April 1982.

2. K. Davis, M. Gold, and D. Makuc, "Access to Health Care for the Poor: Does the Gap Remain?" *Annual Review of Public Health* (Los Angeles: Annual Reviews Inc., 1981), pp. 159–182.

3. See Davis, Gold, and Makuc, "Access to Health Care," for review of literature on access to care of the poor.

4. K. Davis and C. Schoen, *Health and the War on Poverty: A Ten Year Appraisal* (Washington, D.C.: Brookings Institute, 1978).

5. J. Kleinman, M. Gold, and D. Makuc, "Use of Ambulatory Care by the Poor: Another Look at Equity," *Medical Care* XIX, no. 10 (October 1981): 1011–1029.

6. G.R. Wilensky and D.C. Walden, "Minorities, Poverty, and the Uninsured" (Paper delivered at the 109th meeting of the American Public Health Association, Los Angeles, Calif.) (Hyattsville, Md.: National Center for Health Services Research, U.S. Department of Health and Human Services).

7. J. Hadley, *More Medical Care, Better Health: An Economic Analysis of Mortality Rates* (Washington, D.C.: Urban Institute Press, 1982).

8. M. Grossman and F. Goldman, "The Responsiveness and Impacts of Public Health Policy: The Case of Community Health Centers" (Paper delivered at the 109th meeting of the American Public Health Association, Los Angeles, Calif., November 1981).

9. United States Department of Health and Human Services, Bureau of Community Health Centers, unpublished statistics, *BCRR Reports*, 1980.

10. K. Davis, "Contracting with Community Health Centers," in ed. R. Blendon and T. Moloney *New Approaches to the Medicaid Crisis*, (New York: Frost and Sullivan, 1982).

11. United States Department of Health and Human Services, *BCRR Reports*, 1980.

12. G.L. Glandon and R.S. Shapiro, eds., *Profile of Medical Practice, 1980* (Chicago: American Medical Association, 1980).

13. United States Department of Health and Human Services, Bureau of Community Health Centers, *BCRR Reports*, 1980.

14. M. Freeland, G. Calat, and C.E. Schendler, "Projections of National Health Expenditures, 1980, 1985, 1990," *Health Care Financing Review* 1, no. 3 (Winter 1980): 1–28.

15. H.E. Freeman and G.G. Goetsch, "Use of Community Health Centers: Summary Tables," Institute for Social Science Research, University of California, Los Angeles, September 1980, pp. 1–60.

16. M. Morehead, R. Donaldson, and M. Seravalli, "Comparisons Between OEO Neighborhood Health Centers and Other Health Care Providers of Ratings of Quality Care," *American Journal of Public Health* 61, no. 7 (1971): 1294–1306.

17. Grossman and Goldman, "The Responsiveness and Impact of Public Health Policy."

18. K. Davis, "Reagan Administration Health Policy," *Journal of Public Health Policy*, December 1981.

19. United States House of Representatives, Committee on Energy and Commerce, *Hearings on Medicaid Cutbacks on Infant Care* (Washington, D.C.: Government Printing Office, July 27, 1981).

3

Outpatient Departments: Family Doctor to the Poor?

Charles B. Rangel and
Beverly Birns

The problems of health care in the inner city are unique. In particular, there are problems of access to care, continuity of care, and payment for care for groups that have always been underserved: the elderly, the young, the poor, and the minorities. In New York City, these problems loom very large.

The community with which this chapter is concerned consists of a large proportion of poor black and Hispanic people. In 1978 Harlem/East Harlem was designated as a medically underserved community. Since that time one of the municipal hospitals serving the community has been closed. Harlem is still a medically underserved community. The maternal and neonatal death rate in Harlem is higher than it is in the rest of the city; the death rate from drug use is higher in Harlem than it is in the rest of the city; the homicide rate is higher in Harlem than in the rest of the city; and the number of physicians in private practice is probably lower than in most other metropolitan areas in the country. It has been suggested that more than half of the physician contacts in this community occur in the emergency rooms and outpatient departments (OPDs) of the two municipal hospitals in the area. Harlem today is a medically underserved area, and the topic of how ambulatory care is to be provided is of great importance.

To understand the current status of ambulatory care of the inner-city poor, it is helpful to understand some of the history of health care in the inner cities. As metropolitan areas have increasingly become inhabited by the marginally employed, the unemployed, and the minorities, the white middle class has moved to the suburbs. As the middle class left the cities, the physicians who practiced fee-for-service medicine and some charity care also left. The wealthy continued to pay cash for health care, the middle class has been increasingly provided with health insurance that is employment related, and until the mid-sixties the poor either went to public clinics or received no care at all until they were sick enough to be hospitalized.

Among the factors that led the government to become involved in legislation and health-care funding was the recognition of the fact that during World War II many young men were rejected from the army because of health-related problems. During the sixties, as part of the War on Poverty, Medicaid and Medicare were enacted. By 1980 public programs paid 40

27

percent and private health insurance paid an additional 27 percent of the nation's personal health-care bills.[1] Neither Medicaid nor Medicare ever covered all the health care of the poor, but they did increase the participation of millions of people in the health-care system. These programs have narrowed the gap between health care provided to the middle class and the poor. At this time Medicare is paying less than half of the health expenses of the aged, and further cuts are now being made.

Health Care of Minorities

Blacks and other minorities are disproportionately represented among those whose income is below the poverty level. Health care of minorities, although better than it was in the fifties, is far from satisfactory. A few facts should illustrate this point.

Infant mortality is 100 percent higher for blacks than whites. Black women are far less likely to get prenatal care than whites. In many states Medicaid is available to women only after they have had a baby.

Hypertension is 82 percent higher in black women than in white women.

Lead poisoning is much higher among black children than white children.

Racial differences in care are greatest in metropolitan areas where two-thirds of the white and three-quarters of the black population reside.

Fifteen percent of black compared to 9 percent of white children have never had a physical.

In some poor inner-city New York areas, there is 1 physician for 6,666 people, whereas in affluent areas the ratio is 1 per 500.[2]

New York City, Harlem

Inner-city New Yorkers are the most likely of the U.S. population to depend on hospitals' OPDs and emergency rooms for their care. Last year over 4 million visits were made to New York City's municipal hospitals.[3] Over 500,000 visits were made to Harlem Hospital alone.

Although patients who are cared for as inpatients are in a comparatively modern building, the outpatient clinics are spread out in six buildings. When patients first come to the hospital, they check in at a central registry and then are referred to one of the many clinics. Appointments are made either for nine o'clock in the morning or one o'clock in the afternoon. Block-appointment setting is justified as being time-saving for staff, but it is extremely difficult for patients. In most clinics patients are then taken care of on a first-come, first-served basis. Patients at most clinics are assigned to the "next available physician." The pediatrics department and the high-risk obstetrics department have patients assigned to physicians whom they see on subsequent visits. For most other patients it is unlikely that they have continuity of care, which is both medically and psychologically important.

Who are the physicians? Many of the physicians at Harlem Hospital have been there for many years and are both extremely competent and totally dedicated to patient care. However, several circumstances lead to a high turnover of physicians and also a high percentage of foreign doctors. Even when foreign physicians are as well trained as U.S. physicians, problems in communicating with patients, when a physician's command of the language is poor and the patients are very distressed, increases problems in quality of care.

The quality of patient care is as dependent on the physicians and nurses as it is on the physical facility and the available technology. It is also true that housestaff, the interns and residents, are interested in gaining experience with a wide variety of medical problems as well as having the opportunity to use the most up-to-date technology. Many young physicians therefore select hospitals that have the most current medical technologies over Harlem. However, many of the physicians who do choose to work at Harlem Hospital do so because of their strong commitment to improving the health care of poor minority patients.

Another problem facing Harlem Hospital and other hospitals that serve a disproportionate number of minority patients is the scarcity of black physicians. Although 11.7 percent of the population is black, the percentage of black physicians is 2.4 percent, a fact that is particularly disturbing since minority physicians are more likely to work in medically underserved areas than other physicians. In addition, Meharry Medical School, which has trained 40 percent of the black physicians practicing today, is constantly being threatened by a variety of problems, which will be discussed later.

Another deterrent to good medical care is the lack of a computerized record system. Patients' records are frequently lost, and at times physicians have to order tests to be repeated because the findings have been lost. This not only results in poor patient care but is very wasteful of scarce resources.

If I have painted a somewhat gloomy picture of patient care at Harlem Hospital, I want to make it clear that the hospital is not staffed by uncaring health-care workers in an uncaring community. On the contrary, there are very many dedicated physicians and nurses who devote themselves to the care of their patients. Rather, there is ample evidence that most of Harlem's problems are due to inadequate funding. Although the municipal hospitals were designed to serve the indigent, for many years Harlem Hospital was the only city hospital that served an almost entirely black population. Harlem Hospital was never favored by any administration, and there are many who believe that it was always the last to receive any benefits.

In the sixties the realization that New York had a dual system of medical care— excellent care for the rich and totally inadequate care for the poor— led to many reforms. The first attempt to upgrade the quality of care was to affiliate each municipal hospital with a voluntary hospital or medical school. It was hoped that these affiliations would provide higher-salaried, more qualified physicians as chiefs of staff for the municipal hospitals as well as providing the hospitals with better-trained housestaffs. A second attempt to upgrade health care was undertaken in the establishment of the New York City Health and Hospitals Corporation, whose sole function was the management of all the municipal hospitals.

An affiliation between Harlem Hospital and Columbia University's College of Physicians and Surgeons has brought about some improvements, but patients at Harlem Hospital still do not receive high-quality ambulatory care. At this time new efforts are being made to upgrade patient care by changes in the affiliation contracts. Good ambulatory care requires continuity of care, up-to-date technology, a computerized medical-records system, and a well-trained, dedicated staff. We have discussed Harlem Hospital because we think that the problems faced by inner-city municipal hospitals are more severe than those faced by facilities in other areas. However, at this time it is not only the health of the poor that is in jeopardy.

Where Should We Look for Solutions?

We are currently faced with a crisis in health-care delivery. Each day we hear that the nation cannot afford the ever-increasing costs of hospital care, high-technology medicine, and ambulatory care. In 1981 it is estimated that the United States spent $287 billion for health care, an amount equal to 9.8 percent of the gross national product. Hospital care accounted for 41 percent of total health-care spending. Of total health-care expenditures, 42.7 percent came from public funds. The dollar amounts are staggering.

Although we may not be able to afford what we have been spending, it is not the poor who are making money on Medicaid and Medicare, despite the many media stories on fraud. For many reasons we cannot afford to diminish the care that we provide for the poor. We cannot break promises made to the public. We cannot harm those people who depend on the government for health care. If we must cut costs, we should first establish whether the money that we spend is being well spent. Are we capping the profits that are being made on nursing homes and the new medical technologies? Can we afford to deprive people of care while allowing unlimited profits to accrue to those who invest in "health"?

Good medical care for all citizens requires that we have and continue to support high-technology facilities and the education of physicians to use this technology. We need to have medical centers that have burn units; cardiac-surgery units; hemodialysis units; diagnostic equipment that helps to locate the size and place of aneurisms that are life threatening; and neonatal intensive-care units that sustain the life of newborns. However, there is ample evidence that not all health care should be provided in these high-technology, high-cost facilities. Rather than making patients travel long distances to crowded impersonal clinics in large medical centers, it would seem wiser to expand and support community health centers and community primary-care hospitals. A small, voluntary community hospital may, with the help of philanthropic organizations and some government assistance, become a model for this kind of care. Small hospitals with fewer bureaucratic problems, smaller staffs, smaller waiting rooms and more personal attention may be most adequate for much primary care that occurs in most OPDs and emergency rooms. Community and maternal and child health centers should also be supported as they provide greater access along with the potential for more personal and continuous care.

Prevention

It is undoubtedly true that our best investment of health dollars is in good preventive care and early screening. If we need to choose between spending money on more hospitals and nursing homes or making primary care available to those who are underserved, it seems to me that the answer is quite clear. Early diagnosis and prevention could cut hospital costs enormously.

Early and comprehensive prenatal care is cost effective. Proper nutrition reduces the likelihood of premature birth, and prematurity is one of the major causes of low-birthweight, high-risk infants. We know that by providing pregnant women with adequate care, we cut down on the use of intensive-care nurseries and the long-term costs of mental retardation and physical handicaps associated with low birthweight. Family planning reduces the number of unwanted babies that are born, and genetic screening reduces the likelihood of babies being born with serious diseases that require vast investments of health dollars.

Immunization is one of the best investments of health-care dollars. We need only to remember the days before the polio vaccine when parents lived in dread of their children's getting polio. Polio not only claimed thousands of lives each year but also left thousands of children with life-long handicaps and all-consuming medical bills. Every American child should receive inoculations against all the childhood diseases. We have yet to achieve this goal, and yet immunization funds have been cut.

Screening for hypertension is cost effective. Control of hypertension with diet, exercise, and medication helps prevent strokes, kidney disorders, and heart attacks. All these hypertension-related disorders are extremely expensive to treat when patients require extensive hospitalization and treatment.

Providing mental-health treatment for alcoholics and people with emotional disorders is cost effective. Highway accidents, factory accidents, family violence, and many diseases are related to alcoholism, drug abuse, and mental disorders. Outpatient treatment has been shown to reduce the accidents and problems that lead to expensive hospital and medical costs.

An Ambulatory-Care Model

We believe that more comprehensive and better ambulatory care is needed for the poor in medically underserved areas. The evidence is compelling. People who obtain health care from community health centers get high-quality health care that improves their general health and reduces the necessity for hospitalization.[4] In some states infant mortality and preventable diseases been reduced by more than half. In some studies, hospitalization has been reduced by 25 percent for people receiving health care at community health centers. The annual per-person cost of this kind of primary care is far below the cost in other settings.

Community health centers should be easily accessible so that travel time is minimal. They should have community residents on their boards since the residents are most aware of the problems of their own communities and will also serve as outreach people to inform the community of the services available. Staffs should be well-trained physicians committed to primary care. In addition to physicians, the centers should use health-care teams that include nurse practitioners and physicians' assistants. Many activities usually performed by physicians can be performed as well or better by these other qualified health-care workers, and at a lower cost.

Setting appointments at specified times rather than block appointments would facilitate patient care and avoid long waiting periods. Hours should also be set in the evenings and on weekends to accommodate the needs of workers or families with several children. This kind of scheduling would reduce the use of emergency rooms for care that does not require special procedures as well as expand access for those who cannot make appointments between nine and five o'clock.

Close cooperation is required between community health centers and the nearest medical center so that when hospitalization or high-technology procedures are required, the transfer is simple and information exchange is complete. All medical records should be computerized so that complete records for every patient are always available. Eliminating repetition of procedures due to lost or unavailable records would result in vast monetary savings. Community-health-center physicians should have admitting privileges at the hospital to provide for the maximum possible continuity of care. Good health care can be both humane and cost efficient.

Cost Containment

The kind of care just described should be available to those who have neither the cash nor the job-related insurance to cover visits to private physicians. While access to care is crucial, it is possible to spend less for health care by being sure that health dollars are spent wisely. The amount of money that poor people pay for health care should not be increased because that will only result in less care and ultimately in greater costs. Currently Medicare covers less than 44 percent of the health costs of the elderly, and Medicaid never covered more than 33 percent of the cost for the poor. These funds must be protected. However, methods such as prospective reimbursement, outpatient minor surgery, caps on nursing-home rates and hospital-reimbursement rates can reduce costs. Another cost-saving device would be the expansion of home health-care services. Many of the elderly could be maintained in their own homes, with the services of visiting nurses, aides, and physicians, for considerably less than is spent on nursing-home care. Tax deductions could be given to families who take care of their elderly relatives at home.

Conclusions

Our needs are very great. We need individual initiative. At Harlem Hospital we have that, as illustrated by the case of a nurse who has worked for years with hemodialysis patients. Being sensitive to the problems faced by these patients, she initiated a voluntary group of patients who chose the format of a club. This club has been meeting every month. At Christmas and Thanksgiving, there is a party for the club members. The patients discuss their illness, families, friends, diets, medical care, and the hardship of dialysis; and they discuss how best to cope. A current study of the records of these patients, comparing them to hemodialysis patients who have not had this group experience, indicates that the patients in the club enjoy better health and live longer than patients not in the club.

We need leadership and dedication. At Harlem Hospital and other inner-city hospitals, we do have that. At Harlem the chiefs of staff of pediatrics and obstetrics have under very difficult conditions established caring, efficient services that reflect good medical practice. The perinatal mortality figure at Harlem Hospital has dropped from about 25 per 1,000 births to 9 per 1,000 and is now lower than the rest of New York City.

We need help from the private sector, however, who, because of their commitment but not obligation, can help to evaluate programs and also offer assistance to hospitals interested in developing innovative programs. We also need help from the government. Health-care programs and funding were established to eliminate the gap between the excellent care received by the wealthy and the inadequate care received by the poor. The gap has narrowed, but equality of care has not yet been established.

This is a very difficult time for those of us who have spent years trying to establish good health care for all our citizens. We are presently witnessing cuts in funding for Medicaid and Medicare, two programs that have improved the health care of the nation's poorest people—the young, the old, and the minorities. It is terrible to think about patients' being denied admission to hospitals when they are critically ill or when they have been in accidents because the hospitals fear that they will not be paid. It is terrible to think about deregulating nursing homes and turning the clock back to the dismal conditions that originally led to the regulation of the nursing-home industry.

We need to continue to struggle to defend federal support for health care. We also have to wage all the smaller battles as we confront them. Even in these difficult times we are winning some of them. One of these battles concerns Meharry Medical College, mentioned earlier in this chapter. Although the school is crucial to the increase in numbers of black physicians, it nearly lost its accreditation when the accreditation committee determined that its students did not have sufficient access to patients to learn clinical medicine. Meharry had tried unsuccessfully for years to establish a training affiliation with a Veterans Administration hospital in Nashville. The Congressional Black Caucus asked the president for help, and he appointed a task force that recommended short- and long-range solutions. These measures are being taken, and Meharry has retained its accreditation. Thus black physicians will continue to be trained and available to provide needed primary care to underserved areas with large minority populations.

Notes

1. United States Department of Health and Human Services, *Health— United States*, 1981, prepublication copy.

2. Institute of Medicine, *Health Care in the Context of Civil Rights* (Washington D.C.: National Academy Press, 1981); and United States Department of Health, Education and Welfare, *Health Status of Minorities and Low Income Groups*, 1980.

3. Carol Bellamy, *The Health and Hospitals Corporation: Family Doctor to More than Half of New York*, New York: Office of the City Council President, April 1982.

4. Karen Davis, Marsha Gold, and Diane Makuc, "Access to Health Care for the Poor: Does the Gap Remain?" *Annual Review of Public Health* 2(1981): 159.

**Part II
The Payers' Perspective**

4 The Medicare and Medicaid Perspective

George J. Schieber

This chapter discusses the basic issues surrounding payment for ambulatory-care services from the perspective of the federal health-care-financing programs, Medicare and Medicaid. First, the Medicare and Medicaid programs are described. Second, historical and current expenditure patterns are analyzed. Third, the problems in current Medicare and Medicaid ambulatory-care payment practices are discussed. Fourth, the issues that will need to be addressed in reform of the programs are enumerated.

Medicare and Medicaid

Medicare

Medicare is a federal health-insurance program for the aged and disabled. It covers approximately 29 million aged and disabled people. Private insurance companies act as fiscal agents, performing most claims processing and administrative functions. Medicare outlays in FY 1983 will be $57 billion.[1]

Medicare consists of two parts, a Hospital Insurance Program (Part A) and a Supplementary Medical Insurance Program (Part B). All people sixty-five or older who qualify for social-security cash benefits and people who have been receiving social-security disability benefits for twenty-four months or more are automatically enrolled in Part A. Part A is financed by a 2.6-percent payroll tax shared equally by employers and employees. It covers ninety days of inpatient hospital care per spell-of-illness and allows an additional sixty days to be used over the beneficiary's lifetime (for example, lifetime reserve days). Part A also covers one hundred skilled-nursing-facility days per spell-of-illness and an unlimited number of home health visits. Inpatient hospital services are subject to a deductible (currently $260) per spell-of-illness. There is also coinsurance for days 61–90 of inpatient hospital care (one-fourth of the deductible), for each of the sixty lifetime reserve days (one-half of the deductible), and for days 21–100 of skilled-nursing-facility care (one-eighth of the deductible).

Under the Medicare program, hospitals, skilled-nursing facilities and

---

The views expressed in this paper are those of the author. No official support or endorsement by the U.S. Department of Health and Human Services is intended or should be inferred.

home health agencies are reimbursed based on the reasonable cost of covered services furnished to program beneficiaries. These costs are determined through a process of cost allocation and cost apportionment. Essentially, the costs of a hospital's non-revenue-producing cost centers, or overhead costs (depreciation, housekeeping, and so on), are *stepped-down*, or allocated, to the hospital's revenue-producing cost centers (routine, x-ray, outpatient department, lab, and so on). The overhead costs are stepped down using some prescribed or agreed-upon basis of allocation. For example, depreciation might be allocated based on the relative proportion of square feet in each department, and housekeeping might be based on hours of service.

After the allowable direct and indirect costs of the revenue-producing cost centers are determined, these costs are then apportioned between Medicare and other users of the institution. Routine costs (room, board, and nursing) are apportioned on a per-day basis, that is, total routine costs are divided by the total routine days, and the resulting per-day cost is multiplied by the number of Medicare patient days. The costs of an intensive-care unit (ICU) or other special-care unit are also apportioned on a per-day basis. The costs of the ancillary services (x-ray, pharmacy, and so on) are apportioned on the basis of the relative proportion of Medicare charges to total charges for that activity, broken down by inpatient, outpatient, and any subprovider category (for example, a hospital-based, skilled-nursing facility). The ultimate result of this process is that outpatient hospital, other nonroutine, and nonspecial care-unit services are reimbursed on the basis of the proportion of Medicare charges to total charges for these services, multiplied by their costs.

Medicare, by statute, is required to establish limits on the reasonable costs for which it will reimburse. Currently Medicare limits hospitals' routine per-day costs to 108 percent of the group mean of comparable hospitals, skilled-nursing facilities' routine per-day costs to 112 percent of the group mean, and home-health-agency visit costs to the seventy-fifth percentile. Hospitals and other Part A service providers must accept Medicare reasonable cost reimbursements as payment in full. Additional billing of beneficiaries is generally not permitted.

Medicare Part B benefits are available on a voluntary basis to the disabled enrolled in Part A and to all individuals over sixty-five who pay the monthly premium ($12.20 as of July 1982). Premiums finance about one-quarter of program costs, with the remaining three-quarters coming from general revenues. Part B covers physician services, OPD services, home health services, laboratory services, and so on. These services are all subject to a $75 annual deductible and 20 percent coinsurance.

While hospital OPDs and home health agencies are reimbursed on the basis of the reasonable-cost principles just discussed, physicians and other

Part B practitioners are paid on the basis of their customary, prevailing and reasonable (CPR) charges. A physician's (or other Part B practitioner's) reasonable charge for a particular medical procedure is the lowest of his actual billed charge, his customary charge, and the prevailing charge (that is, the charge generally made by other physicians for the same service in that particular geographic area).

Customary and prevailing charges are calculated from statistical formulas using physicians' charges to Medicare in the previous calendar year. Separate prevailing charges are generally established for different specialties and geographic areas. Increases in Medicare prevailing charges are limited to increases in an economic index, reflecting increases in office-practice costs and general earnings levels in the economy. Physicians and other Part B practitioners can bill beneficiaries for amounts in excess of the program-determined reasonable charges.

Medicaid

Medicaid is a state-administered, federal-matching-grant program that finances medical services for certain categories of low-income people, primarily those eligible to receive cash payments under (1) the Aid to Families with Dependent Children (AFDC) program and (2) the Supplemental Security Income (SSI) program for the aged, blind, and disabled. In addition, some thirty states have exercised the option of extending coverage to "medically needy" people who meet the SSI or AFDC categorical criteria but whose incomes are slightly above the welfare standards or who have incurred substantial medical expenses. An estimated 22 million people are Medicaid recipients. States may process claims themselves or contract with private organizations. The federal share of the program is financed from general revenues. On the average, the federal share is about 55 percent but ranges from 50 percent in the highest-per-capita-income states to 77 percent in the lowest-per-capita-income states. Federal and state Medicaid outlays in FY 1983 will be about $36 billion, of which the federal government will pay $19.9 billion.[2]

Federal law mandates that states cover inpatient and outpatient hospital, physician, skilled-nursing-facility, family-planning, home health, laboratory, x-ray, rural-health-clinic, and nurse-midwife services for all eligible recipients, and early and periodic screening, diagnosis, and treatment (EPSDT) services for children under twenty-one. States may also provide a variety of optional services including intermediate-care-facility services, dental services, prescription drugs, and clinic services. States may limit the amount, duration, and scope of services. Coinsurance may be imposed only in limited instances, and the amounts must be nominal.

States have considerable discretion in establishing reimbursement methods and rates. For hospitals and nursing homes, states must establish rates that are consonant with efficient operation. A 1982 survey showed that thirty-two of the state Medicaid programs (of fifty responding) used Medicare cost principles to reimburse for inpatient hospital care. For OPD services, most states have adopted Medicare reimbursement principles. In 1982 thirty-three states (of 47 responding) used Medicare reasonable-cost principles to pay for OPD services while fourteen used fee-schedule or prospective-payment approaches. For the physician component of ambulatory services, however, most states have developed their own reimbursement procedures. While most Medicaid practitioners are reimbursed on a fee-for-service basis, only fourteen states (of forty-seven responding) used the Medicare CPR approach; twelve used some variant of the Medicare CPR method; twenty used fee schedules; and one used a relative-value scale.[3] Providers who participate in the program must accept Medicaid-determined reimbursements as payment in full and cannot bill beneficiaries.

Expenditure and Use Trends

Analyzing the levels and trends in ambulatory-care spending under Medicare and Medicaid is problematic. Since Medicare and Medicaid cover specific service types such as physicians, inpatient hospitals, outpatient hospitals, drugs, and so on, program data are collected for these basic service types but not an amalgam called "ambulatory care." Under Medicare the bulk of ambulatory-care spending is for physicians and hospital outpatient services. Under the Medicaid program, significant expenditures are also made for drugs, dental care, eyeglasses, and other health services and supplies.

Table 4–1 contains information about Medicare, Medicaid (broken out by federal and state), and total personal-health-care spending for physicians' services, hospital OPD services, other ambulatory services, and all services for fiscal years 1970 and 1980. The physician data include both inpatient and outpatient physician expenditures. Since consistent time-series data on inpatient versus outpatient physician spending are not readily available, overall physician-spending trends are analyzed. Unpublished Medicare data indicate that about 60 percent of Medicare physician reimbursements are for inpatients. Unpublished Medicaid data show that between 20 to 25 percent of all Medicaid physician visits were for inpatients. Applying these percentages to the 1980 data in table 4–1 indicates outpatient physician spending of about $3.0 billion for Medicare and $1.7 billion for Medicaid. Thus overall Medicare ambulatory-care spending in 1980 was about $5.8 billion, 17 percent of all Medicare spending, while Medicaid

Table 4-1

Medicare, Medicaid, and Total Personal-Health-Care Spending by Type of Service

Type of Service	Medicare (Millions of Dollars)	Percent of Total	Medicaid (Millions of Dollars)	Percent of Total	Total Personal (Millions of Dollars)
FY 1970					
All services	6,783	11.1	4,613	7.6	60,866
Physician services	1,616	11.9	590	4.4	13,524
Outpatient hospital[a]	93	5.4	189	10.9	1,736
Other ambulatory[b]	61	0.4	715	4.5	15,810
FY 1980					
All services	33,938	16.1	25,781	12.3	210,299
Physician services	7,452	16.5	2,261	5.0	45,059
Outpatient hospital[a]	1,910	19.3	1,102	11.1	9,914
Other ambulatory[b]	886	2.0	2,568	5.6	44,165

Source: Robert M. Gibson and Daniel R. Waldo, "National Health Expenditures, 1980," *Health Care Financing Review* (September, 1981); supplemented with unpublished data, Bureau of Data Management and Strategy, Health Care Financing Administration, U.S. Department of Health and Human Services.

[a]"Outpatient hospital" includes expenditures on end-stage renal disease facilities, rural health clinics, and on minor amounts of other Part B services. Expenditures on outpatient hospital services per se amount to about 80 percent of the total.

[b]"Other ambulatory" includes eyeglasses and appliances, other health services, drugs and medical sundries, and dentists' services.

ambulatory-care spending was about $5.4 billion, 21 percent of all Medicaid expenditures.

The share of total personal-health spending devoted to physician and hospital outpatient services has changed little between 1970 and 1980, accounting for about one-quarter in both years. (If "other ambulatory" is included, these services accounted for about one-half of all personal-health-care expenditures in both years.) Nevertheless, there was significant growth in spending on these as well as all on other health services. Between 1970 and 1980, total overall physician-services spending increased by 235 percent from $13.5 billion in 1970 to $45.1 billion in 1980, while overall spending on outpatient hospital services increased by 470 percent from $1.7 billion to $9.9 billion. Over this same period total personal-health spending increased by 245 percent from $60.9 billion to $210 billion.

There have, however, been substantial increases in spending as well as shifts in the Medicare and Medicaid shares of total physician- and out-patient-services spending. This is especially true for Medicare OPD services. These expenditures increased from $93 million in 1970 to $1.9 billion in 1980, a 1,950-percent increase. Medicare's share of total OPD services spending increased from 5.4 percent in 1970 to 19.3 percent in 1980. As a percentage of Medicare spending, hospital outpatient expenditures increased from 1.4 percent in 1970 to 5.6 percent in 1980. While Medicaid's share of OPD spending remained about the same, at 11 percent, actual spending increased 485 percent from $189 million in 1970 to $1.1 billion in 1980. As a percentage of Medicaid spending, hospital outpatient expenditures increased slightly from 4.1 percent in 1970 to 4.3 percent in 1980. Largely due to Medicare, the Medicare and Medicaid share of all hospital outpatient-services expenditures increased from 16.3 percent in 1970 to 30.4 percent in 1980.

Medicare and Medicaid physician-services shares and spending have exhibited similar, albeit less sensational, growth. Medicare physician-services expenditures increased by 360 percent from $1.6 billion in 1970 to $7.5 billion in 1980. Medicare's share of total physician spending increased from 11.9 percent to 16.5 percent. Physician expenditures accounted for 23.8 percent of 1970 Medicare spending compared to 22.0 percent in 1980. Medicaid physician spending increased by 285 percent from $590 million in 1970 to $2.3 billion in 1980, while the Medicaid share of total spending increased slightly from 4.4 to 5.0 percent. Physician spending under Medicaid accounted for 12.8 percent of all Medicaid spending in 1970 and 8.8 percent in 1980. The combined Medicare and Medicaid share of physician-services expenditures increased from 16.3 to 21.5 percent.

Increases in Medicare and Medicaid physician- and outpatient-services expenditures are due to increased numbers of people using services, increases in the prices of services, and increased intensity/use per person. Unfortunately, there are no reliable data to separately measure the price and use/intensity factors. Nevertheless, in understanding the increases in expenditures for these services, it is instructive to examine use patterns. Table 4–2 contains Medicare and Medicaid data for fiscal years 1970 and 1980 on the number of users of services and per-user expenditures.

The number of Medicare beneficiaries using reimbursed outpatient services increased by 315 percent, from 1.8 million in 1970 to 7.2 million in 1980. (This compares to only a 40-percent increase in the overall number of Medicare beneficiaries.) Some of this increase is attributable to more beneficiaries' meeting an essentially fixed Part B deductible (the deductible was increased from $50 to $60 in 1972), while hospital outpatient costs increased steadily throughout the period.[4] However, Medicare expenditures per user of services increased by 410 percent, from $50 in 1970 to $256 in 1980. This increase reflects both increases in price and use/intensity of services.

Use of outpatient services by Medicaid beneficiaries also increased significantly. The number of beneficiaries using services increased by 160 percent from 3.7 million in 1970 to 9.6 million in 1980. (This compares to a 49-percent increase in Medicaid beneficiaries.) Per-user expenditures in-

Table 4-2
Use and Cost per User for Medicare and Medicaid Physician and Outpatient Hospital Services

Use and Cost	Medicare		Medicaid	
	1970	1980	1970	1980
Physician-services				
users (in thousands)	8,189	16,841	9,747	13,762
Reimbursements per user	$203	$470	$58	$136
Outpatient-services				
users (in thousands)	1,750	7,237	3,706	9,578
Reimbursements per user	$50	$256	$51	$115

Source: Unpublished data from Bureau of Data Management and Strategy, Health Care Financing Administration, U.S. Department of Health and Human Services.

creased by 125 percent from $51 in 1970 to $115 in 1980, significantly less than the Medicare increase.

The number of Medicare beneficiaries using reimbursed physician services increased by 105 percent, from 8.2 million in 1970 to 16.8 million in 1980. As before, much of this increase results from more beneficiaries' meeting the fixed Part B deductible.[5] Per-user physician expenditures increased by 130 percent from $203 to $470. For Medicaid the number of users of physician services increased by 40 percent from 9.7 million in 1970 to 13.8 million in 1980. Per-user expenditures increased by 135 percent from $58 to $136.

It is hard to draw any definitive conclusions from these data. Medicare users of hospital outpatient and physician services and expenditures for these services increased at far higher rates than did comparable figures for Medicaid. A large portion of the Medicare increases can be attributed to the coverage under Medicare in 1972 of the disabled and those with end-stage renal disease. Nevertheless, data on aged Medicare beneficiaries indicate a 260-percent increase in the number of aged users of outpatient hospital services (6.3 million in 1980) and a 270-percent increase in per-aged-user expenditures ($186 in 1980). Similarly, the number of aged users of physician services increased by 85 percent (15.1 million in 1980), and per-user expenditures increased by 120 percent ($451 in 1980).[6]

The increased number of users of services due to growth in the respective beneficiary populations as well as changes in Medicare and Medicaid eligibility rules account for a substantial part of the increase in physician and outpatient hospital expenditures. Increases in the prices of services and the number and intensity of services per user also account for large portions of these expenditure increases. The openended reasonable cost and charge-reimbursement systems used by Medicare and Medicaid provide few financial incentives to limit costs and charges, nor do they provide incentives to promote the appropriate number, type, and place of service.

Medicare and Medicaid
Ambulatory-Care-Reimbursement Problems

Medicare- and Medicaid-reimbursement practices should encourage high-quality medicine, efficiency in the health-care-delivery system, participation of medical-care providers, access to care for program beneficiaries, and administrative simplicity. Current Medicare- and Medicaid-reimbursement practices for ambulatory care (as well as institutional care) fall short of achieving these policy goals.

Physician Reimbursement

Medicare physician-payment practices have not encouraged efficiency on a number of grounds. First, both Medicare fees and Medicare physician expenditures have increased at highly inflationary rates. Second, Medicare-payment practices have resulted in unwarranted specialist-reimbursement differentials for physicians performing the same service; payment imbalances that favor high technology, diagnostic, laboratory, and surgical procedures; inhospital treatments instead of ambulatory-based care; and higher urban than rural payments, even after adjusting for cost-of-living differences.[7] These incentives inherent in current Medicare physician-payment practices are counter to public-policy objectives of encouraging additional physician time over unnecessary procedures, primary over tertiary care, and outpatient instead of inpatient care. They also tend to reinforce physicians' decisions to locate in urban rather than rural areas.

Perhaps the worst feature of the current Medicare-payment system is that it is rapidly becoming a series of specialty-specific, local fee schedules set at the prevailing-charge level. This system exists because prevailing charges are limited by the economic index, while customary and actual charges are unconstrained. Thus an increasing number of actual and customary charges exceed the prevailing charge, which then essentially determines the reasonable charge. As a result, all the undesirable urban-rural, specialty, and other reimbursement imbalances in the present system are being locked into place.

The present Medicare-payment system does not encourage physician participation or financial protection for beneficiaries since physicians can decide on a claim-by-claim basis whether to accept the Medicare reasonable charge as payment in full, known as "accepting assignment," or whether to require the beneficiary to pay the full actual-billed amount. When the physician accepts assignment, he submits the bill to the Medicare program and agrees to accept the Medicare reasonable charge less the requisite beneficiary cost sharing as payment in full. When physicians do not accept assignment, they bill the beneficiary directly, and Medicare reimburses the beneficiary the reasonable charge less the requisite cost sharing. The beneficiary is responsible for any difference between the physician's actual-billed charge and the Medicare reasonable charge.

While the assignment rate (that is, the percentage of claims on which physicians accept assignment) has been relatively stable (at about 50 percent) over the past eight years, the percentage difference between actual charges and Medicare reasonable charges has almost doubled over this time period. For example, in 1973 actual charges were on average 12 percent higher than Medicare reasonable charges, while in 1981 they were 23 percent higher. As a result, for the 50 percent of unassigned claims, beneficiaries are facing substantially larger out-of-pocket costs. The Medicare-payment system is also complex and costly to administer and is confusing to beneficiaries and physicians. Neither beneficiary nor physician knows what Medicare will reimburse until the claim is actually paid.

The problems with Medicaid physician-reimbursement practices are somewhat different. Those state Medicaid programs that follow Medicare principles and/or base payments on physicians' actual charging patterns suffer from the same problems just discussed. However, the basic problem with Medicaid physician-reimbursement practices is that in many states payment rates are so low that physicians do not participate in the program. For example, in 1980 Medicaid-payment rates were less than 80 percent of the Medicare levels in twenty states for general practitioners and twenty-six states for specialists.[8] Since physicians must accept Medicaid reimbursement as payment in full, many physicians will not see Medicaid patients. This results in beneficiaries being forced to seek care in more expensive hospital inpatient or outpatient settings. This is clearly counterproductive in terms of both cost containment and continuity of care.

Outpatient Reimbursement

Medicare-payment practices for outpatient care do not encourage efficiency and are complex to administer. Many of the problems with Medicare outpatient-reimbursement procedures pertain to both the general use of and the specific implementation of the Medicare reasonable-cost reimbursement principles. Reasonable-cost reimbursement generically provides few incentives for efficiency. As the expenditure data presented earlier indicate, Medicare payments for outpatient hospital services have been increasing at rapid rates.

Furthermore, Medicare reimbursements for outpatient services are unlikely to reflect real resource costs and hence do not encourage an efficient allocation of resources. This inaccuracy occurs for several reasons. First, since there is no standard definition of an outpatient visit or outpatient case mix, neither hospitals nor the federal government can accurately equate incurred costs with real resource use. Second, determining Medicare outpatient reimbursements on the basis of a ratio of charges to Medicare patients divided by gross charges to all patients times costs is unlikely to result in reimbursement approximating real resource costs since the hospital's charge structure is essentially a construct that is designed to maximize revenues. Third, since Medicare limits inpatient routine costs but not ancillary or outpatient costs, hospitals have incentives to shift costs to ancillary or outpatient cost centers. Fourth, rules used to allocate costs among non-revenue- and revenue-producing cost centers—as well as apportionment of costs among cost centers and payors—are likely to cause costs to be arbitrarily shifted to the outpatient setting. Fifth, the plethora of compensation and billing arrangements used by hospital-based physicians also often leads to the hospital billing for the physicians' services and inexact allocations of costs and charges between the physician and hospital.[9]

Other problems in Medicare ambulatory-care reimbursement occur because physicians practicing in hospital OPD settings are reimbursed separately and on a different basis from the hospital. Thus physicians practicing in hospital settings have few incentives to restrain costs by limiting use of hospital resources since all reasonable hospital costs are reimbursed by Medicare. A second problem concerns the reasonable charges of physicians practicing in hospital outpatient settings relative to those of office-based physicians. Currently, hospital-based and office-based physicians face the same prevailing charges. About 40 percent of the prevailing charge represents office overhead costs. Physicians practicing in hospital OPD settings bear no overhead costs since Medicare reimburses the hospital for all nonphysician, outpatient hospital costs. Therefore, paying physicians practicing in the hospital OPD at a rate that includes the overhead costs of office-based practices results in duplicate payment of overhead costs.

The effects of Medicaid hospital outpatient-service-reimbursement policies are similar. In the states using the Medicare-reimbursement system, many of the preceding problems are germane to Medicaid. However, in those states using fee schedules or other prospective payment methods for hospital outpatient reimbursement, other problems may occur. To the extent that fees are less than the hospitals' costs, hospitals may be discouraged from treating Medicaid patients. If they continue to treat such patients, inadequate payment levels may promote financial distress. Inner-city, public, general hospitals with large numbers of Medicaid patients would be the most severely hurt. Furthermore, if both physician and outpatient payment rates are low, access for Medicaid beneficiaries may be impeded. To the extent that these beneficiaries then require hospitalization for more serious medical problems, overall costs would increase.

Reform Issues

Future federal reforms will to a large extent depend on basic administration health-policy directions. Competitive market forces could obviate the need for federal regulation. On the other hand, to the extent that a federal Medicare program persists and that efforts to federalize Medicaid reach fruition, federal involvement in reimbursement will continue. Moreover, legislation enacted by Congress in 1981 requires establishment of limits on both the physician and hospital components of hospital outpatient services.

Reimbursement reforms in the ambulatory-care area are dependent on reforms in the institutional-care setting. Rationalization of ambulatory-care reimbursement to promote efficiency would probably not achieve overall systems savings if hospitals continue to be reimbursed on a reasonable-cost or a charge basis. Moreover, efforts by the federal government to promote efficiency may not produce significant overall systems savings if other payors do not follow suit.

Nevertheless, federal efforts to reform current physician and hospital outpatient-reimbursement practices will have to deal with several issues. On the physician side, fee schedules have proven less inflationary than CPR and could be established to eliminate many of the problems inherent in the current CPR system. Nevertheless, many difficult issues remain.

Among these are how the schedules would be established; would they be set by government or physicians, by negotiations, or by relative-value scales? How would relative values be established? Who would represent physicians? At what geographic aggregation would schedules be established? Would the schedules apply only to Medicare and Medicaid, to all federal programs, or to all payors? Would there be separate schedules for different specialties? How would "specialists" be defined? What type of physician-participation system would be employed? Could physicians extra-bill beneficiaries? How would medical procedures be defined for reimbursement purposes? What constraints, if any, would there be on use? Could incentives be established to encourage physicians to be cost-conscious case managers? Would overall expenditures be limited?

Issues surrounding hospital outpatient-reimbursement reform are equally formidable. How would the unit of service be defined? How would differences in case mix among hospitals and other ambulatory-care settings be measured? How do hospital inpatient case mixes relate to outpatient case mixes? How can resource inputs be accurately measured? How can the cost be measured for stand-by time, medical education and joint inpatient and outpatient products? On what bases can outpatient hospital costs be compared to other ambulatory-care settings? What accounting and reporting procedures are needed to assure consistent measurement? To what extent do physicians influence outpatient and inpatient hospital-resource use?

These questions illustrate the complex issues requiring some resolution in any broad initiative to provide incentives for efficiency in Medicare and Medicaid. In the meantime the substantial cost increases in Medicare and Medicaid are taxing the ability of the federal government to provide services to the aged and poor. While there is never enough information to make completely informed public-policy choices, it is important that policies promote genuine reforms rather than merely limit federal liability or shift cost to beneficiaries, state governments, or other payors.

Notes

1. United States Department of Health and Human Services, *The Fiscal Year 1983 Budget Press Release* (Washington, D.C.: Department of Health and Human Services, February 8, 1982).

2. Ibid. and Donald N. Muse and Darwin Sawyer, *The Medicare and Medicaid Data Book, 1981* (Washington, D.C.: U.S. Department of Health and Human Services, 1982).

3. LaJolla Management Corporation, "Volume 1 Medicaid Program Characteristics Summary Tables," unpublished preliminary draft (Rockville, Md.: LaJolla Management Corporation, April 1982).

4. United States Department of Health, Education and Welfare, Social Security Administration, *Medicare: Health Insurance for the Aged, 1969, Section 1: Summary: Utilization and Reimbursement by Person* (Washington, D.C.: Social Security Administration, 1975), and Unpublished Data, Bureau of Data Management and Strategy.

5. Ibid.

6. Unpublished Data, Bureau of Data Management and Strategy, Health Care Financing Administration. See also Raymond L. Goldsteen, *Medicare: Use of Hospital Outpatient Services, 1979* (Washington, D.C.: Health Care Financing Administration, 1981).

7. See Ira L. Burney, et al., "Medicare and Medicaid Physician Payment Incentives," *Health Care Financing Review* (Summer 1979) (Washington, D.C.: Health Care Financing Administration).

8. See John Holahan, "A Comparison of Medicaid and Medicare Physician Reimbursement Rates," Discussion paper (Washington, D.C.: The Urban Institute, 1982).

9. For discussions of some of these issues, see Marsha Gold, "Hospital-

Based Versus Free-Standing Primary Care Costs," *Journal of Ambulatory Care Management*, February 1979, and Stuart Altman et al., *Ambulatory Care: An Analysis of Costs in Alternate Settings* (Waltham, Mass.: Brandeis University Health Policy Consortium, 1980).

5 The Blue Cross and Blue Shield Perspective

Neil Hollander and
David Ehrenfried

One of the central topics of the discussion in this book is the cost of ambulatory care and the appropriate use of hospital outpatient services. Common concerns are that these services are often used when physician office or other less expensive services could have been used instead, that hospital outpatient services are often priced too high, and that third-party payers and the public in general are therefore paying more than they should for ambulatory care.

Blue Cross and Blue Shield Plans, as major payers of ambulatory care, figure prominently in this controversy. Along with the practices of Medicare, Medicaid, and other third-party payers, those of Blue Cross and Blue Shield Plans are frequently accused of fostering the use of more expensive health-care services, or discouraging the use of less expensive ones. It is said that third-party benefit-and-payment policies influence health-care choices by covering high-cost (hospital) services more favorably than low-cost (physician office) alternatives. There is a strong sense, therefore, that Blue Cross and Blue Shield Plans ought to be concerned about the costly ramifications of these alleged practices and should pursue steps to modify them.

As a matter of policy, the Blue Cross and Blue Shield organizations are concerned about the ways in which ambulatory care is delivered and reimbursed. The opening sentence of the Blue Cross and Blue Shield Association's recent policy on ambulatory surgery states that "surgery, like any other health care service, should be performed in the least costly manner enabling delivery of safe, high quality patient care."[1] The policy also identifies specific steps Blue Cross and Blue Shield Plans should take to promote this principle, including the revision of benefit-and-payment policies that may discourage reasonable substitution of less expensive for more expensive services. It also acknowledges that in addressing benefit-and-payment practices related to the cost of ambulatory care, Blue Cross and Blue Shield Plans face many complex practical issues.

Concerns that certain Blue Cross and Blue Shield Plans may be overpaying for ambulatory care have to be tempered by a number of factors, not the least of which is an overriding goal to reduce inpatient-care costs. Providing outpatient coverage is seen as one way of accomplishing that. Given the enormous costs of hospital inpatient care, it may be reasonable to

53

risk and, for the time being, to accept some overuse or overpayment for ambulatory-care services. Aside from this consideration, it should not always be assumed that hospital outpatient services are necessarily more expensive than other ambulatory alternatives. Neither is it always clear that plan benefits are really as influential in the choice of care as some believe or that certain changes in benefit structure and payment policies will necessarily affect such choices.

This chapter is devoted to discussing these issues. But first, some background on the development of Blue Cross and Blue Shield coverage for ambulatory care is useful.

Development of Ambulatory-Care Coverage

Blue Cross and Blue Shield Plans began covering outpatient services early in their development. From their inception in the 1930s and 1940s, most Blue Shield Plans (or "medical-service plans," as they were originally known) covered surgeon's services in physician offices as well as in hospitals. A small number of plans also provided benefits for physician medical services delivered in the office and in the home. Most Blue Cross Plans, which also were founded in the 1930s and 1940s to pay for hospital inpatient services, routinely covered hospital emergency-room services by the end of World War II, although many covered such care in the 1930s as well. One of the primary objectives of both types of coverage was to provide Blue Cross and Blue Shield subscribers with affordable and reasonable access to these ambulatory services.

Even during their early years, those who were administering the plans were conscious of the potential for abuse and overuse. Coverage generally excluded routine medical care and often placed strict limits on the amounts that would be reimbursed for each service and during each enrollment period.[2] It was recognized quite early that responsible underwriting of prepaid health coverage requires balancing the goal of facilitating access to care against the fiscal conservatism necessitated by the limited control third-party payers have over use.

During the 1950s and 1960s, the plans expanded hospital outpatient benefits considerably. Steadily rising personal income and increased competition from commercial insurers made outpatient coverage an increasingly attractive benefit to underwrite. Minor hospital outpatient surgery was an early addition, and by the mid-1950s a number of Blue Cross and Blue Shield Plans were experimenting with benefits covering outpatient diagnostic laboratory and x-ray services. During the same period many Blue Shield Plans also added benefits for office diagnostic services. These diagnostic-service benefits were almost always subject to per-visit or yearly limits and were usually purchased in the form of policy or benefit riders to the basic package of hospital inpatient benefit and medical-surgical benefits. A further development during this period was the broad introduction of supplemental major-medical benefits, which frequently covered office medical (as opposed to surgical) care.

While adding outpatient diagnostic benefits, a number of Blue Cross and Blue Shield Plans also excluded benefits for diagnostic inpatient admissions. Despite these policies, the plan administrators were often skeptical about the potential for substituting outpatient for inpatient diagnostic services. The plan administrators that studied the introduction of outpatient diagnostic benefits during those years concluded that, on balance, outpatient diagnostic benefits added at least as much to cost through increased use as they saved through foregone admissions.[3] Plan policymakers were also sensitive to the pros and cons of applying different cost-sharing and other limits on outpatient benefits to influence the use and actuarial value of these benefits. In fact, considerable discussion among plan administrators took place in developing the precise level and scope of outpatient-care benefits that would be offered for such groups as the federal employees, the automobile companies, and other major Blue Cross and Blue Shield customers.

Over the past twelve years, plans have introduced outpatient benefits at an increasingly rapid rate. Not only have the number of groups and individuals with such coverage increased to include almost all Blue Cross and Blue Shield subscribers, but coverage has been made more comprehensive as well. The trend has been to make coverage for outpatient surgery, diagnostic and therapeutic services, and emergency care comparable to that for similar services provided on an inpatient basis. Annual dollar limits and the like have frequently been dropped when they did not also apply to inpatient benefits. At the same time major medical benefits covering office medical care have become ubiquitous in group programs. A number of Blue Cross and Blue Shield Plans also began offering benefit programs to cover preventive services such as regular check-ups and other routine care.

A major impetus for recent expansion in ambulatory-care coverage has been great concern over health-care-cost inflation. Overall Blue Cross and Blue Shield Plans have reacted by taking steps designed to reduce inpatient use. It thus became increasingly important for plans to provide avenues for outpatient substitution for inpatient care while simultaneously applying pressures on inpatient care through utilization review, payment changes, and public education, on the one hand, and limits on outpatient care through benefit restraints, on the other.

Growth in Use of Outpatient Facilities

Partly as a result of the steps just described, the use of outpatient care by Blue Cross and Blue Shield members has increased dramatically. The Blue

Cross and Blue Shield Associations commissioned an independent study of Blue Cross and Blue Shield use trends. Preliminary results from the study lend support to the theory that there are strong relationships between the efforts to decrease member use of inpatient services, the decline in their use of such services, and the increase in the use of outpatient services. In 1947, the first year for which there is national Blue Cross data on outpatient care, there were approximately ten outpatient visits per 1,000 members. By 1957 the rate more than doubled to twenty-three visits per 1,000, and by 1961, the rate had increased to sixty visits per 1,000.

Over the next two decades, the outpatient-visit rate continued to increase significantly. At the same time Blue Cross inpatient-admission rates decreased. The outpatient-visit rate was 165 per 1,000 members by 1971, a 175-percent increase over the 1961 rate. By 1981 the rate had grown to 353 per 1,000, a 114-percent increase over the rate ten years earlier. Meanwhile the inpatient-admission rate for Blue Cross members decreased nearly 10 percent over the 1971–1981 period from 125 admissions per 1,000 members in 1971 to 113 per 1,000 in 1981. The patient day rate decreased roughly 20 percent from 891 days per 1,000 members in 1971 to 717 per 1,000 in 1981. Overall, there were three times as many outpatient visits as inpatient admissions in 1981, compared to only one-third more in 1971.

In dollar terms, average Blue Cross payments per outpatient visit nearly doubled from $42 to $77 per visit in just the five years from 1976 to 1981. Altogether, outpatient care now represented about 12 percent of all Blue Cross benefit payments in 1981 compared to about 8.5 percent five years earlier.

For a variety of reasons, information on the growth in Blue Shield benefits paid for physician services performed in ambulatory settings is not as good as for Blue Cross benefits. However, our experience indicates that the Blue Shield trend toward greater use of benefits for ambulatory care is essentially similar.

Perspective on Growing Ambulatory-Care Costs

Given the enormous growth in the amount and cost of ambulatory care, Blue Cross and Blue Shield Plans are concerned that perhaps much of this care may be unnecessary, too expensive, or rendered in inappropriate settings. However, it must be stressed again in this regard that the big picture for the plans is the continued great use and high cost of inpatient services. The cold fact is that the plans pay roughly ten times more for inpatient care than for outpatient care. It therefore makes sense for Blue Cross and Blue Shield Plans to focus their main efforts on reducing reliance on inpatient care and to emphasize outpatient care as one of its logical and less costly substitutes. In this context one can perhaps risk being a little simplistic and look favorably on increasing ambulatory-care expenditures as long as the use of more costly inpatient alternatives continues to decline.

In any case, Blue Cross and Blue Shield Plans fully expect to pay more for ambulatory care. Not only is the quantity of ambulatory care provided continuing to increase but ambulatory care is growing qualitatively more complicated and sophisticated. These qualitative changes, in particular, help raise the average unit costs of ambulatory care due to the increased intensity and elaborateness of the services being rendered. Yet because these changes appear to reflect increasing substitution of outpatient for inpatient care, larger payments for ambulatory care are often viewed as a positive trend.

Issues in the Cost of Ambulatory Care

The preceding statements notwithstanding, it is generally acknowledged that some ambulatory care received by Blue Cross and Blue Shield members may be more expensive than it ought to be. Some Blue Cross and Blue Shield patients undoubtedly use hospital emergency rooms and outpatient clinics when they could visit less costly physician offices. However, econometric studies by Sloan, Cromwell, and others suggest that this is not nearly so large a practice for patients with private health insurance as it is for those without such coverage.[4] Additional support for this proposition is provided by a small survey done in 1977 by Blue Cross of Massachusetts. That survey indicates that most plan members who went to emergency rooms did so because their physicians were not available, because they had no regular physicians, or because no other reasonable alternative was available. In any case over the past ten years a number of Blue Cross and Blue Shield Plans, such as those in Michigan, Wisconsin, Cleveland, and Washington, D.C., have responded to large increases in emergency-room use by tightening benefit criteria used in paying benefits for this care and by screening emergency-room claims more closely.

Surgery is another area where outpatient-facility settings are sometimes used when less expensive office settings would be equally safe and convenient. For example, information on vasectomies collected from a number of Blue Cross and Blue Shield Plans in different parts of the country demonstrate significant variations in where the surgery is performed, that is, in physicians' offices or outpatient facilities. The percentage of such procedures performed in offices ranged from 47 to 86 percent in different plan service areas. A number of plan administrators view such variation as a source of concern and are taking steps to address it, including physician-education programs and increased payments for certain office-based surgery.

One such plan is Blue Cross and Blue Shield of Arizona. The Arizona plan found, after examining its own claims records, that a number of surgical procedures that could have been done in the office had been done instead in hospital and freestanding ambulatory-surgery units. Discussions with Arizona surgeons indicated that these facilities were considered convenient and that there was sometimes little incentive to perform certain procedures in their offices. Since physicians were reimbursed the same amounts regardless of the setting in which they performed surgery, it was evident some physicians felt it advantageous to use hospital and freestanding facilities, particularly since the facilities seemed better able to capture surgical overhead expenses. In an attempt to change some of the financial incentives, the plan administrators decided to try paying surgeons an additional amount for a selected number of procedures when performed in the office. Over thirty other Blue Cross and Blue Shield Plans have or are planning similar programs. So far these programs are too new to allow us to know if they are having the desired effects on costs and use, although efforts are underway to evaluate them in a number of locations.

Blue Cross and Blue Shield Plans are also concerned about other factors that tend to escalate ambulatory-care costs. These include poor provider management, unfavorable provider pricing policies, and various benefit or reimbursement restrictions. With regard to poor management, health-care providers often have higher costs than necessary. The U.S. General Accounting Office recently documented wide variations in the prices providers pay for laboratory, drug, and other services.[5] A recent article in the *Journal of the American Medical Association* on the overordering of emergency-room services provides evidence that hospitals can substantially decrease the number of emergency-room laboratory and drug charges through vigorous efforts to identify and reduce unnecessary use of these services.[6]

The fact that these and other inefficiencies are so apparent in the delivery of care poses a dilemma for third-party payers. There are limits on the extent to which payers can affect the day-to-day operations or practices in hospitals and doctors' offices. Attempts to dictate how care should be delivered, even if that were possible, are not very palatable; among other things, they are expensive to administer, confusing, and often quite inequitable. Other less direct approaches must generally suffice. For instance, programs for monitoring and controlling the use of ambulatory services—especially ancillary services—may have some impact. Changing productivity incentives through different payment mechanisms may also hold promise. Preferred-provider organizations, capitation, and certain forms of prospective reimbursement may also help create incentives for providers to be more efficient. Even simple reductions in payment amounts may have some positive effects, although this approach could eventually reduce access to care, if not also its quality. Arbitrary pay reductions could also create considerable ill-will with Blue Cross and Blue Shield accounts and sub-scribers since they would be the ones who would inevitably bear the brunt of provider discontent with such measures. In the final analysis, inefficiencies in the delivery of health care can be remedied only by health-care providers themselves, although that does not mean payers will not try increasingly aggressive remedies of their own to solve persistent problems.

Unfavorable pricing of ambulatory services is another difficult problem. There seem to be mixed findings and opinions on the subject of whether certain providers have different costs that would justify different payment levels. It is well established that health care is generally less costly when provided in a physician's office than when provided in a hospital. However, studies such as those done by several Blue Cross and Blue Shield Plans, by the Health Care Financing Administration, and by the Greater New York Hospital Association provide contradictory evidence about whether hospi-tal outpatient care is more expensive than comparable care delivered by freestanding ambulatory-care facilities.[7,8]

The price and cost differences between hospital and freestanding set-tings may often be elusive in the sense that hospitals are often able to manipulate their costs and charges. One description of how this is possible is provided in a study of Medicare-cost reporting done for the Robert Wood Johnson Foundation Ambulatory Care Cost Project. That study shows that ambulatory-care costs can be manipulated by hospitals in determining Medicare-reimbursement levels.[9] The use of budgeting procedures by hos-pitals to manipulate outpatient-service prices, even to the extent of making them comparable to physician office charges, is discussed in a seldom-cited 1970 Rand Corporation study by Taylor and Newhouse.[10] In any case, hospitals do seem able to exercise discretion in this area, for a number of Blue Cross Plans have observed that hospitals do sometimes lower OPD charges when faced with stiff competition from freestanding facilities.

Another factor that can affect the pricing of ambulatory services is third-party-payment practices. Historically, plan administrators have based payment for these services on providers' charges. Today about two-thirds of the Blue Cross Plans base reimbursement for outpatient services on charges (compared to less than half that do so for inpatient services). While paying on the basis of charges need not result in plan administrators' reimbursing amounts that are unfair to their subscribers, it can present problems if providers succeed in inflating these charges to make up for revenue short-falls associated with insufficient or slow payment from other sources or to settle unmet financing requirements associated with costs not related to providing services to Blue Cross subscribers. In such cases Blue Cross and Blue Shield Plans ought to be concerned that their subscribers may be subsidizing services delivered to others. Given that Blue Cross and Blue Shield coverage of ambulatory services is usually broad and comprehensive, it is unfair for Blue Cross and Blue Shield Plans to pay the same charges that are billed for other patients with less extensive coverage or slow and inefficient payers.

A final issue that needs to be discussed is whether Blue Cross and Blue Shield benefit-and-payment practices encourage proper use of ambulatory services. A criticism often heard in this regard is that traditional benefit-and-payment policies promote use of more costly ambulatory-care services.

Taking a historical perspective again, most Blue Cross and Blue Shield benefits for ambulatory services are motivated by complex and changing social and business forces. These benefits can anticipate health-care-delivery trends to a degree, but for the most part, they trail health-care demand that has been made apparent by such factors as clinical developments in medicine, changing patient preferences, collective-bargaining decisions, and general economic conditions. Consequently, today's benefits reflect a highly variable combination of factors: namely, what health-care providers *thought* should be delivered; what subscribers and employers *thought* was important to cover; and, finally, what insurers *thought* could be reasonably underwritten.

Decision making in this context has been, and still is, a dynamic process. The results of this process, especially as they affect cost and use, have always been subject to reevaluation and change. Thus more and more Blue Cross and Blue Shield Plans are performing utilization review of outpatient services to help control and redirect inappropriate use. Many are also offering incentives to physicians and other health-care providers to promote the selection of economical health-care settings.

Importantly, there is a sense that plans can do more to improve the delivery and cost of ambulatory care. Much of the emphasis is understandably on promoting substitutes for inpatient care. Some emphasis is also on finding cost-effective ways to cover routine or preventive medical services. Thus the range of plan responses includes increased development of health-maintenance organizations (HMOs) and increased coverage of primary care such as the Pioneer Benefit Program in New Jersey and the Pediatric Preventive Health Maintenance Program in Pennsylvania. Others, like the California Blue Shield Health Incentive Program, give individual subscribers cash incentives as motivation for reducing their use of health-care services. Still other approaches, like the Blue Cross experiments to reimburse hospitals on a per capita basis in North Dakota and Massachusetts, should help encourage providers to improve outpatient services by increasing incentives for them to render care more efficiently.

In conclusion, the Blue Cross and Blue Shield perspective on paying for ambulatory care is shaped by the overwhelming need to contain the rising costs of inpatient care. Covering ambulatory care is an essential part of that effort. However, as the cost and use of ambulatory services increase, the same ingenuity applied to containing inpatient services will have to be applied in the ambulatory arena as well.

Notes

1. Blue Cross and Blue Shield Associations, "Policy and Recommendations of the Blue Cross and Blue Shield Association on Ambulatory Surgery" (Chicago: January 1981).

2. Louis S. Reed, *Blue Cross and Medical Service Plans* (Washington, D.C.: Federal Security Administration, 1947).

3. Mary Ann Steep and Thomas J. Tilley, "Outpatient Diagnostic Benefits and the Effects of Inpatient Experience: A Three Part Study," *Inquiry* II, no. 1 (June 1965): 3–12; Denwood Kelly, "Experience with a Program of Coverage for Diagnostic Procedures Provided in Physicians' Offices and Hospital Outpatient Departments," *Inquiry* II, no. 3 (December 1965): 28–44; and Daniel Hill and James E. Veney, "Kansas Blue Cross–Blue Shield Benefits Experience," *Medical Care*, March–April 1970, pp. 143–158.

4. Frank Sloan, Jerry Cromwell, and Janet Mitchell, *Private Physicians and Public Programs* (Lexington, Mass.: D.C. Heath-Lexington Books, 1978); Frank Sloan and Judith Bentkover, *Access to Ambulatory Care and the U.S. Economy* (Lexington, Mass.: D.C. Heath-Lexington Books, 1979); and Victor Fuchs and Marsha Karmer, *Determinants of Expenditures for Physicians' Services in the United States, 1948–1968* (Washington, D.C.: National Center for Health Services Research and Development, 1972).

5. United States Comptroller General, *Hospitals in Same Area Often Pay Widely Different Prices for Comparable Supply Items* (Washington, D.C.: General Accounting Office, 1980).

6. Steven Karas, Jr., M.D., "Cost Containment in Emergency Medicine," *Journal of the American Medical Association* 243, no. 13 (April 4, 1980): 1356–1359.

7. Donald Orkand, et al., *Comparative Evaluation of Costs, Quality and System Effects of Ambulatory Surgery Performed in Alternative Settings, Final Report* (Washington, D.C.: U.S. Department of Health, Education and Welfare, 1977).

8. *Ambulatory Care: An Overview and Comparative Analysis of Hospital Based and Freestanding Delivery Systems* (New York: Greater New York Hospital Association, 1979).

9. David Young, Elinor Socholitzky, and Edward Locke, "Ambulatory Care Costs and the Medicare Cost Report: Managerial and Public Policy Implications," *The Journal of Ambulatory Care Management* 5, no. 1 (February 1982): 13–29.

10. Vincent Taylor and Joseph P. Newhouse, *Improving Budgeting Procedures and Outpatient Operations in Non-profit Hospitals* (Santa Monica, Calif.: Rand Corporation, 1970).

6

A State Perspective

Robert M. Crane and
Edward S. Salsberg

Ambulatory-care services of the highest quality, accessible to all people at reasonable cost, must be the cornerstone of any health-care-delivery system. A number of factors have made this goal difficult to achieve in New York State, despite a strong commitment to it on the part of state government. While some encouraging initiatives have been taken to address some of the difficult ambulatory-care issues, the prospects for the future are not bright, particularly in light of reductions in federal commitments and programs and state financial constraints. The state's goals and objectives for ambulatory care include: access to quality ambulatory care, particularly primary care, for all state residents; efficient and varied ambulatory-care-delivery systems; containment of costs; and an integrated regulatory system to meet these goals including standards for quality care, reimbursement, and certification of need.

While New York State and health-care providers have been moving consistently and steadily toward achievement of these goals, many problems still exist. The delivery system, in some parts of New York State, is dominated by high-cost providers; this discourages access for the poor and near poor. There are a significant number of state residents who lack adequate income and insurance to pay for ambulatory care. Many providers serving the poor and near poor are facing severe financial difficulties that may increase costs and decrease access. Finally, the system does not effectively encourage expanded access, efficiency, or cost containment.

The first section of this paper reviews some of the major problems the state faces regarding paying for ambulatory care. The second section reviews New York State's activities to address these problems. Possible future developments, both at the state and federal level, which may affect reimbursement for ambulatory care, are reviewed in the last section.

Payment Issues in Ambulatory Care

Ambulatory-care services in New York are characterized by a number of features that must be taken into account in solving problems of ambulatory-care financing and costs. In terms of numbers of providers, ambulatory care constitutes the single largest and most important component of the health-care system in New York.[1] Yet it remains the least understood and controlled element of the health-care system. The inadequate attention that is often paid to this component by policymakers is due in part to the fact that in terms of current state expenditures, ambulatory care represents a relatively minor cost component compared to hospital and long-term-care expenditures.

Institutions, particularly teaching hospitals and municipal hospitals, are a major source of ambulatory-care services in New York State. This is especially true for Medicaid recipients and residents of medically underserved communities.

In addition, these institutions are providing a growing number of ambulatory-care services to populations with special needs such as mental-health and methadone-maintenance services. However, despite the number and diversity of ambulatory-care services and providers in New York State, primary-care services are not available to all residents.

Institutional ambulatory care is costly to provide. Existing funding and third-party coverage for these services, particularly for the poor, are inadequate. As a result, institutions providing ambulatory-care services in underserved communities have incurred significant deficits. Finally, there currently are significant gaps in our knowledge of where ambulatory-care services are rendered, to whom, at what relative costs, and the appropriateness of alternative settings. These issues are explored in detail in the following pages.

Reliance on Institutional Ambulatory-Care Providers

New York State's ambulatory-care system is critically dependent on institutional providers, particularly in communities with shortages of physicians in private practice. Nearly one-third—24 million of the state's 75 million—ambulatory-care visits are made to institutional settings, including hospital OPDs, emergency rooms, and freestanding ambulatory-care centers.[2] In New York nearly 22 percent of all visits are to hospital OPDs and emergency rooms compared to 12 to 15 percent nationally.[3]

Institutional providers are often the only significant source of ambulatory care in many low-income communities. This reflects a number of factors including the paucity of noninstitutional providers in these communities, the greater accessibility because of their hours of operation, and their willingness to provide service regardless of an individual's ability to pay. For many reasons there has also been a significant decline in private practicing physicians in many of these communities. For example, in New York City the number of general practitioners in office-based practice has declined 50 percent in the last ten years.[4]

Medicaid beneficiaries and low-income people are especially dependent on institutional providers. In New York City, Medicaid recipients represent only about 17 percent of the population, but 43 percent of the hospital-based visits.[5,6] This in part reflects the locations of the institutional providers in primary-care-shortage areas. Approximately 17.5 percent of the state population live in these areas, yet 31 percent of all institutional visits and 38 percent of all hospital OPD visits are in shortage areas.[7]

Among institutional providers, hospitals, as opposed to freestanding clinics, provide the majority of institutional ambulatory services: Of all institutional visits in 1979, 69 percent were to hospitals.[8] In addition, the vast majority of hospital visits are in New York City, which accounted for 63 percent of all hospital-based ambulatory-care visits and 78 percent of all Medicaid, hospital-based, ambulatory-care visits in the state.[9]

It should also be noted that in New York City, teaching institutions and the municipal hospitals play a very important role. Fifty-one OPDs, those operated by thirteen municipal hospitals and thirty-eight teaching hospitals in New York City, furnish 62 percent of all outpatient visits in the state.[10] New York City is a national resource for medical education and training, with twice as many medical students and three times as many physicians in training as would be expected for its population.[11] Statewide, over 26 percent of all patients in teaching hospitals are Medicaid recipients, compared to about 11 percent in non-teaching hospitals.[12] While the exact impact of medical education and training on the use and costs of services is not clear, it is recognized as a factor in the increased cost of care. New York City municipal hospitals are also a major provider of hospital-based ambulatory-care services; in 1978 they provided 32 percent of the state's OPD visits.[13]

This heavy reliance on institutional providers creates a number of problems for the state as well as for individuals. Hospital OPDs are often inappropriate settings for primary care, and care is often fragmented and uncoordinated. Yet many Medicaid beneficiaries and medically indigent rely on hospitals for primary care. While we lack conclusive data concerning the relative cost of care in different settings, adjusted for case mix, it appears that ambulatory care provided in the hospital setting is more expensive than other settings, particularly for primary care. In addition, there is a higher use of ancillary services and inpatient services.

The Medicaid Program and Ambulatory Care

The state's largest tax-levy expenditure for health services, including ambulatory care, is through the Medicaid program. Nevertheless, as table 6–1 illustrates, ambulatory-care services represent a relatively small share of total state Medicaid expenditures.

Table 6-1
New York State Medicaid Expenditures by Type of Service,
Fiscal Year 1979/80

Type of Service	Millions of Dollars	Percent
Inpatient hospital	992	30
Skilled-nursing facility	1,037	32
Intermediate-care facility (general and MR)	259	8
Hospital ambulatory-care services	232	7
Freestanding ambulatory-care clinics	98	3
Physician (inpatient and ambulatory)	121	4
Dental	50	2
Drugs	108	3
All other	397	11
Total	3,294	100

Source: New York State Health Planning Commission, in conjunction with New York's health and human-services agencies, *New York State's Medical Assistance Program: A State Handbook*, February 1982.

Despite the relatively small share of Medicaid expenditures that go to ambulatory-care services, these services are used by a high percentage of Medicaid recipients. For example, in New York City, 63 percent of the recipients used physician services that accounted for only 4 percent of the expenditures, and 36 percent used hospital outpatient clinics that accounted for 7 percent of the expenditures.[14]

Medicaid Rate Setting

In the mid-1960s when Medicaid was first introduced, New York State had generous eligibility standards, and large numbers of New Yorkers became eligible for the program. By 1968, however, the cost of the program far exceeded the state's original projections. Beginning in 1969, the state undertook a series of measures designed to reduce Medicaid costs. Eligibility levels were sharply reduced in 1969 and 1971, and today they remain lower, in absolute dollar terms, than they were in 1966. In addition, physician fees were reduced. No effort, however, was made to directly control reimbursement for institutional ambulatory-care services. Facilities were reimbursed on an all-inclusive, prospectively set rate based on total reported costs without limitations. A cost per visit, based on the most current cost report, was calculated and trended forward for inflation, to establish a rate for the coming year.

Despite these cutbacks, Medicaid costs continued to rise, especially for institutional-based, ambulatory-care services. The prospective-reimbursement methodology, in place from 1970 to 1975, contained no efficiency standards or ceilings. During this period, Medicaid expenditures for institutional ambulatory-care providers rose threefold. In 1976 when New York City and New York State were facing their most serious financial crisis, further cutbacks in the Medicaid program became necessary. In light of the rapid rise during the prior years and the preference to modify reimbursement rather than reduce benefits or eligibility, institutional ambulatory-care reimbursement was sharply limited beginning in 1976. Subsequent years saw further changes:

In 1976 Medicaid rates for OPDs, emergency rooms, and diagnostic-and-treatment centers were frozen at 1975 rates.

In 1977 the freeze continued and a $50 rate ceiling was added.

In 1978 rates were allowed to increase 5 percent over 1977 rates, but the $50 ceiling was continued.

In 1979 the $50 ceiling was continued but was applied only to the operating component of the rate, which was allowed to increase 5 percent, up to the $50 ceiling. All capital costs were included in the rate, thus permitting the actual final rate to exceed $50.

In 1980 the methodology changed substantially. The base year was updated to 1978, and the cost per visit was trended to 1980. The ceiling on operating costs was increased to $55, and capital costs were again passed through and included in the rate.

In 1981 the base year was updated (to 1979), and the operating cost ceiling was increased to $60 with the capital component added to the rate.

Rates for freestanding facilities, known as diagnostic-and-treatment centers (or D&Ts), in New York State were held to the constraints just outlined from 1976 to 1979. In 1980 a multistep methodology using cost-based-peer-group ceilings was introduced in the rate-setting process. Diagnostic-and-treatment centers were divided into eleven service-related peer groups such as multiservice centers, family-planning clinics, methadone-maintenance treatment programs, hemodialysis, and rehabilitation clinics. Within each group, the 1977 reported allowable costs for each facility were used to calculate a weighted-average rate per visit. Group ceilings, set at 105 percent of the weighted average or the 1977 reported allowable costs, whichever was lower, were trended to 1980 to establish a facility's rate. The same methodology, with 1978 as the base year, was used to set the 1981 rates.

As noted earlier, physician fees were reduced in 1969 in an effort to reduce Medicaid expenditures. They were later restored to their original 1966 level, where they remained until August 1980, when office-visit fees for primary-care practitioners were increased by an average of 18 percent. Other physician fees remain unchanged.

During the last decade, there were a number of changes, external to the Medicaid-reimbursement policies, that complicate interpretation of the impact of these policies. For example, in addition to the more stringent Medicaid reimbursement, the state also instituted stricter eligibility screening. As a result, the number of people eligible for Medicaid decreased 15 percent (355,000 persons) from 1975 to 1979.[15]

As indicated in table 6–2, Medicaid OPD visits increased slightly from 1978 to 1980, and total Medicaid costs rose sharply in 1980, primarily reflecting the increase in the average reimbursement rate and some growth in the number of visits. Most interesting is the sharp rise in the cost per visit and the increase in the difference between the Medicaid rate and the cost. This may reflect a shift in cost allocation within the hospital. Beginning with the ambulatory-care rate freeze in 1976, there was an incentive to shift reported costs into inpatient cost centers. As the controls began to loosen in 1979 (with the capital pass-through) and in 1980, there may have been an incentive to shift costs to ambulatory-care cost centers.

Visit trend data for the last decade do not reflect a significant change in Medicaid use of hospital ambulatory-care services although the figures

Table 6–2
Trends in Hospital Outpatient Department Services

Year	Total OPD Visits (Thousands)	Medicaid OPD Visits (Thousands)	Estimated Medicaid Expenditures (Millions of Dollars)	Estimated Average Medicaid Rate per Visit (Dollars)[a]	Estimated Cost per Visit (Dollars)	Difference in Rate and Cost per Visit (Dollars)
1978	8,063	3,008	128.7	42.79	54.04	11.25
1979	7,878	3,091	148.8	47.15	57.84	10.50
1980	8,588	3,154	180.0	56.14	63.07	6.93
1981			194.0	61.37	74.06	12.69

Sources: New York State Department of Health, Internal Documents; New York State Office of Health Systems Management, *Preliminary Report to the Legislature on Ambulatory Care*, September 1979; New York State Office of Health Systems Management, *Final Report to the Legislature on Ambulatory Care*, January 1980; New York State Office of Health Systems Management, *Report to the Legislature on Ambulatory Care Reimbursement*, January 1981; and New York State Office of Health Systems Management, *1982 Report to the Legislature on Ambulatory Care Reimbursement*, January 1982.

Note: "Hospital outpatient department services" includes only "all-inclusive clinics" and excludes emergency rooms and specialty clinics.

[a]Medicaid rate years coincide with the state's fiscal year, April 1 through March 31.

reflect some growth in the visits per person given the drop in people covered by Medicaid.

While institutional-based ambulatory-care reimbursement has been constrained for the last seven years, physician fees have been even more limited since the start of the program. The result is that relatively few physicians in private practice participate in the Medicaid program to any significant degree.

One of the results of the current environment, including the reimbursement policies, is the development of numerous shared health facilities, better known as "Medicaid Mills." While the number in New York has decreased during the last four years (since the state increased its monitoring efforts), they remain an important source of care in many inner-city areas. Few individual physicians could afford to establish a private practice in an inner-city area and rely on the Medicaid fee schedule and the medically indigent. Shared health facilities appear to be an entrepreneurial phenomenon that has succeeded by relying on the provision of routine care to a high volume of Medicaid patients, limited service to medically indigent patients, and referral of difficult cases to institutional providers.

The Medically Indigent

The medically indigent are generally those people whose incomes or resources are too high for Medicaid eligibility but who lack sufficient funds to purchase health insurance. This group also includes many people who have insurance but whose coverage is limited to inpatient care and who cannot afford to pay for high-cost ambulatory-care services. These people often use hospital emergency rooms, municipal-hospital OPDs, local health-department clinics, and neighborhood health centers.

A 1980 Department of Health and Human Services (DHHS) study estimated that 8.8 percent of New York State residents lacked health insurance.[16] This number may have grown since 1980, due to the continued recession.

Institutional Ambulatory-Care Deficits

Serious financial problems face some institutional providers, particularly those in underserved low-income areas. Ambulatory care is a major source of such facilities' deficits. The total operational deficit reported for voluntary hospitals in 1978 was $247 million, $167 million of which was for hospital ambulatory-care services. In addition, the New York City municipal hospitals, probably the largest source of care for the medically indigent, estimated that $209 million in tax-levy subsidies was required to make up the difference between costs and revenues for ambulatory-care services in FY 1978/79.[17] Local health departments and community health centers also receive considerable direct tax-levy support for the provision of ambulatory-care services.

These deficits are created by a number of factors. First, there are a large number of self-pay/no-pay users. The medically indigent often find that institutional providers are their only possible source of care. As shown in table 6–3, the self-pay users represent a significant percentage of the ambulatory-care patients at both hospitals and D&Ts.

Many facilities use a sliding-fee schedule and charge the medically indigent based on their income. Often the charge is only a few dollars, and self-pay collections are generally very limited.

Second, Medicaid's reimbursement policies have sought to contain program costs and encourage efficiency. Even with an average Medicaid reimbursement of over $61 for hospital clinics in 1981, facilities have been unable to keep costs within the limits of approved rates, and deficits have resulted. Third, poor management and the structure of traditionally organized OPDs result in fragmented care, inadequate control of costs, excessive use of ancillary services, the mixing of teaching and training with the

Table 6–3
Distribution of Visits by Payer Source in New York State, 1979
(percent)

Payer Source	Outpatient Departments	Emergency Rooms	Diagnostic and Treatment Centers
Medicaid	39.2	20.2	40.2
Medicare	14.2	7.9	5.2
Blue Cross	2.5	24.1	.7
All other	44.1	47.8	53.9[a]
Total	100.0	100.0	100.0
Distribution of all other[b]			
Workman's compensation	0.3	5.9	
Commercial insurance	4.1	5.7	
Self-pay	25.8	22.6	
Free care	2.7	1.6	
Other	11.2	12.0	
Total	44.1	47.8	

Source: New York State Council on Health Care Financing, *Preliminary Report on Ambulatory Care*, March 1982.

[a]This includes considerable direct state- and federal-grant funds.

[b]Not collected for diagnostic and treatment centers. Not all OPD's and ER's answered the detailed breakdown for "all other." The percentages shown here have been normalized by converting to 100 percent and then to the base percent for all OPDs and ERs. This has resulted in minor changes in percents but no change in the relative relationship among payer sources.

delivery of services, and poor cost-allocation techniques. These practices have led to increased costs and poor collections.

State Response

New York State is probably more involved with ambulatory-care delivery and providers than most other states. This reflects the state's longstanding commitment to assuring access to primary care. This concern has led the state to undertake a wide range of programs and activities, as well as provide extensive financial support for ambulatory care. These efforts have been aimed at both the delivery system and the financing mechanisms.

The overall strategy of the state includes three major objectives: (1) to provide direct support for ambulatory-care services to the medically indigent through grants to health providers; (2) to establish a regulatory and reimbursement framework that promotes efficient delivery of services; and (3) to provide funding and support for demonstration projects in the delivery and financing of ambulatory-care services.

Some of the specific programs and efforts supported by the state are described in the following paragraphs.

The Ghetto Medicine Program

This program, initiated in 1968, provides funding for ambulatory-care services to the medically indigent. To receive funding under this program, health facilities must meet certain minimum standards in terms of the organization of services. These standards are intended to help assure an adequate quality of care as well as access to care for the medically indigent.

The Blue Cross Ambulatory-Care-Service Loss

State legislation requires that third-party payors include, as an inpatient cost, the net loss incurred by a voluntary hospital in rendering ambulatory and emergency services. Medicaid and Medicare do not currently participate. Blue Cross, however, does include ambulatory-care losses in the calculation of Blue Cross inpatient rates.

Categorical and Public-Health-Support Programs

The state provides support to an array of categorical and local-health-department programs. This includes, for example, grants to health providers for hypertension control, maternal and child health, and family-planning services.

The Primary Ambulatory-Care Program (PACP)

The PACP was initially authorized and funded by the legislature in 1978 for the initiation, development, and study of mechanisms for expanding and improving the quality of primary ambulatory-care services, particularly for the medically indigent and other residents of underserved areas.

Demonstration Projects

In addition to the PACP projects, the state is actively involved in a number of other projects that affect the financing and delivery of ambulatory-care services. The Bedford-Stuyvesant/Crown Heights demonstration, for example, receives extensive state and federal support for three hospitals and two freestanding health centers in Brooklyn which serve low-income residents. One of its goals is the reorganization of ambulatory-care services in the community. The Metropolitan Hospital has another demonstration that includes major reforms at the hospital, a new coverage category for the medically indigent enrolled at the hospital (Citycaid), and the development of a case-management system at the hospital.

Technical Assistance

The state has provided technical assistance to a number of communities seeking to expand the availability of primary ambulatory-care services. This has led to a number of community health centers' receiving state and/or federal support.

Future Directions for New York State

As indicated by the preceding efforts, New York State is committed to maintaining and improving the availability of ambulatory-care services, particularly primary-care services. Yet the reimbursement policies that have saved the Medicaid program and all other payers billions of dollars have contributed to the fiscal instability of many providers. We must now look ahead and institutionalize in our regulatory and reimbursement systems the supports and incentives to strengthen ambulatory care while assuring its availability at reasonable cost.

New York State recognizes that to contain the long-run cost of health care, we must develop and maintain effective primary ambulatory-care services for all residents regardless of income. Unfortunately, the recent federal cutbacks go in the opposite direction. Programs supporting health care, particularly primary care, have been cut sharply. This has the potential of reversing progress made in expanding access over the past decade.

Partly as a result of federal policy, the current environment is extremely challenging: access to care, particularly quality primary care, is still a problem for many; some health facilities in underserved areas are facing serious financial problems; the federal government is reducing its commitment and funding for ambulatory-care programs; and the state budget is severely strained by the recession and the decrease in federal program support.

We need to target our efforts and funding to assure that our priorities are addressed. Thus, we have adopted these strategies for ambulatory care in the 1980s.

1. *Stabilization of the hospital sector as a major provider of ambulatory care through the development of a restructured hospital-reimbursement methodology.* New York State recently received approval from the federal Health Care Financing Administration (HCFA) to implement an innovative three-year hospital inpatient-financing program incorporating uniform prospective-reimbursement methodologies for all third-party payors including Medicaid, Medicare, and Blue Cross; a guaranteed three-year revenue cap trended for inflation; and allowances for bad debt, charity care, and discretionary purposes. The proposal reflects nearly three years of discussions and negotiations, among the state, the legislature, providers, and insurers.

Under this new program, each hospital payer will be required to add a factor to its rate that will be pooled and distributed to hospitals experiencing deficits caused by bad debts and charity care. Eligibility for the funds will depend on each facility's effort to obtain payment from those it serves and the continuity of effort in providing services to patients unable or unwilling to pay.

The total state resources available to finance bad debt and charity care will average 3 percent of total state-reimbursable costs over the next three years. The funds will be distributed to a hospital based on its ambulatory and inpatient bad debt and charity care. Because of these added allowances for bad debt and charity care incorporated into the new reimbursement proposal, the Blue Cross Ambulatory Service Loss (ASL) allowance and part of the state-funded Ghetto Medicine program will be eliminated.

An additional quarter of a percent of total state-reimbursable costs will be made available on a regional basis annually to avert crises that may threaten an institution's fiscal viability and jeopardize the community's access to quality health care. This proposal will assist hospitals with large ambulatory-care losses resulting from serving large numbers of the medically indigent.

2. *Continuation of the Primary Ambulatory Care program.* The state will continue to support this program and where possible assure that the funds go to the areas of greatest need, as well as to support innovative projects. The PACP will be the major vehicle for assisting freestanding ambulatory-care facilities and will continue to provide direct funds as well as technical assistance. Unfortunately, reductions in federal funding for community health centers may place additional strains on the already limited PACP funds currently available.

3. *Outpatient department reorganization.* The state will explore support of hospital ambulatory-care reorganizations. During the past few years there has been extensive activity and discussion within the hospital industry without state involvement. These reorganizations range from the development of physician-practice plans and other internal-management changes to proposals to separate the OPD from the hospital. Currently we are attempting to identify the key components of reorganization that support our goals, particularly increased access to quality ambulatory care and cost control, while avoiding the unbundling of services only to maximize reimbursement. Yet, given the heavy reliance in New York State on institutional providers, institutional reform is critical.

4. *Change in Medicaid ambulatory-care reimbursement.* Current reimbursement methodologies can become more effective in encouraging cost-effective, quality services. Therefore, the state is involved in a number of demonstrations in institutional reimbursement. One such approach is promotion of capitation reimbursement for both hospitals and community health centers for which we are reviewing specific proposals. Capitation reimbursement, which will include some degree of risk sharing, offers the possibility of rewarding efficiency and substituting ambulatory care for inpatient services. Promoting increased Medicaid enrollment in health-maintenance organizations is one part of this approach. While there are many issues to be addressed, including assurances of access and quality, we are moving forward in this direction.

5. *Freedom of choice, case management, and competition.* The federal Omnibus Budget Reconciliation Act of 1981 permits significant increased flexibility in the state's administration of Medicaid. This includes authority to implement primary-care case-management arrangements to restrict recipients in their choice of providers and to enter into prepaid capitation arrangements with non-HMOs. One proposal from Rochester, approved by the HCFA, would use prepaid capitation and require that all Medicaid recipients select from several comprehensive health-care programs. In general, case management can help assure that services are used effectively and

may help shift use to lower-cost services. The state has set basic principles for proposals which limit freedom of choice for Medicaid recipients, including that projects be convincingly cost effective, assure access to quality ambulatory care, not unduly disrupt recipients and providers, and encourage competition.

6. *The Practitioner Placement program.* New York State has made a significant commitment to medical education, including support of medical students. In return for this support, the state requires a service payback in designated underserved areas. The physicians receiving state support have just recently begun to complete their training. This resource may be a cost-effective source of ambulatory-care services. The Department of Health is expanding its practitioner-placement activities to attract physicians to underserved areas and is also working closely with the National Health Service Corps.

7. *The primary-care profile.* Working with the state's Health Planning Commission, we are developing a primary-care profile to identify those areas with the greatest need for additional health resources. The profile will include a wide range of health-status indicators and health-resources data by primary-care-analysis area—areas defined as rational market and service areas for primary care. Mapping the whole state will permit us to better target our limited resources.

Notes

1. New York State Office of Health Systems Management, *Final Report to the Legislature on Ambulatory Care*, January 1980.
2. New York State Department of Health, *A Working Paper on Outpatient Department Reorganization*, November 1981.
3. New York State Office of Health Systems Management, *1982 Report to the Legislature on Ambulatory Care Reimbursement*, January 1982.
4. United Hospital Fund, *Communities, Hospitals and Health Care: The Role of New York City Hospitals in Serving Their Neighborhood and the Nation* (New York: United Hospital Fund, 1982).
5. New York State Department of Social Services, *Utilization of Health Services by New York City Medicaid Recipients 1979—1980: Program Analysis and Utilization Report 1*, October 1981.
6. New York State Office of Health Systems Management, 1982.
7. New York State Office of Health Systems Management, 1980.
8. New York State Office of Health Systems Management, 1982.
9. Ibid.
10. New York State Department of Health, 1981.

11. United Hospital Fund, 1982.

12. New York State Health Planning Commission, in conjunction with New York's health and human-services agencies, *New York State's Medical Assistance Program: A State Handbook*, February 1982.

13. New York State Office of Health Systems Management, 1980.

14. New York State Department of Social Services, 1981.

15. United Hospital Fund, 1982.

16. Joseph G. Beck and Calvin Pierson, *The Medically Indigent: A State Perspective on a National Problem*, New York State Health Planning Commission, April 1980.

17. Ibid.

Part III
Organizational Considerations
in Ambulatory Care

7 The Role of Hospitals

Linda A. Burns

This chapter focuses on one aspect of ambulatory care, that of physician ambulatory services provided by hospitals, primarily in organized outpatient departments (OPDs), hospital-associated group practices, and emergency departments (EDs). An important question is whether hospital-sponsored or hospital-associated ambulatory-care programs have costs that differ from those for the same services rendered in independent physicians' practices. Its significance lies in the fact that $11.7 billion in revenues were paid to community hospitals in 1980 (excluding payments to physicians) for producing ambulatory care.[1] If costs are higher and quality is the same in the hospital programs as compared to independent programs, sensible public policy would require discouraging the use of hospital programs. If hospital costs are higher and quality is higher, it may be sensible to pay more to hospitals if the quality is worth more than the cost. If costs and quality are the same, reimbursement policy should be neutral regarding the providers of ambulatory care.

Although it is important to determine how quality of services differs among settings, it is not the purpose of this chapter to focus on whether or not quality differences exist. And adequate information is as yet unavailable to answer the question of cost differences among various providers of ambulatory care.

However, in pursuit of this question, two subsidiary questions emerge: What roles do hospitals play in the provision of ambulatory care? How can the cost to hospitals in producing ambulatory care be measured? This chapter will provide a framework for discussing the organization of hospital ambulatory-care programs.

To answer the question about the cost of hospital ambulatory care, an understanding of some of the organizational aspects of ambulatory care and the health industry is necessary. Although much of the information may be common knowledge to health-industry observers, a framework is presented from which discussion concerning ambulatory care and hospitals can ensue.

Types of Ambulatory Care

Ambulatory care provided by or in association with hospitals includes much more than the mere transference of a private physician's practice to the hospital's facilities. The explosion of technology that has transformed health services delivered to patients who are hospitalized has also transformed the patterns of medical practice and services delivered to ambulatory patients.

One way to understand ambulatory care is to envision a spectrum of services ranging from inpatient care to high technology, multidisciplinary care, subspecialty care, primary care, and preventive health services.

The place of any particular ambulatory-care program on the spectrum is determined by the type and number of specialized staff, the mix of medical and health disciplines involved, and the facility and equipment requirements of the programs. Thus on one end of the spectrum is the most technologically sophisticated care such as that rendered by a medical team in a specialized surgical facility with patient-monitoring and life-support equipment.

As one moves along the spectrum, there are other less technological services such as programs requiring the interaction of multidisciplinary teams of physicians, nurses, dieticians, and pharmacists, followed by single-discipline subspecialties. Near the other end of the spectrum would be primary-care services.

Ancillary services such as laboratory tests and radiology procedures should not be confused with physician services. Neither should selected therapies and treatments that can be rendered on an ambulatory basis such as occupational and physical therapies. This chapter thus focuses on ambulatory services provided by physicians.

To state that a hospital provides services to ambulatory patients (that is, patients who are not confined to a bed) conveys little information. The question is, what types of ambulatory services does the hospital provide? In other words, to what extent does the hospital provide high-technology ambulatory services or subspecialty services or primary care? The facility, staffing, and equipment requirements vary considerably depending on the types of ambulatory services a hospital provides. Therefore, meaningful discussion of ambulatory care must rely on a recognition and specification of the types of ambulatory services under review.

Hospital Roles in Ambulatory Care

When speaking of the involvement of any particular hospital in ambulatory care, one must specify the degree of control the individual hospital exercises over the ambulatory-care program. A high degree of control indicates that the hospital has corporate ownership of the program, manages the program, and makes the major policy decisions concerning that particular ambulatory-care program. A low degree of control or involvement is exemplified by a hospital that owns the facility in which the ambulatory-care program resides and leases that facility to health professionals who then operate and manage the program. Hospital-owned physician office buildings are an example of this type of involvement.

The extent to which the hospital controls physician services is critical in determining the degree of control and is relevant to a discussion of hospital ambulatory-care costs. A hospital that hires physicians to provide ambulatory services exercises a greater degree of control than a hospital that does not. However, a hospital that does not have physicians on its payroll may still achieve a high degree of control over its ambulatory-care programs if the hospital is able to place the individual physician or medical group providing services at financial risk through contractual arrangements.

This delineation of hospital roles in ambulatory care leads to the definition of terminology to be used throughout this chapter.[2]

Hospital sponsored. The hospital assumes total fiscal and legal accountability for the ambulatory-care programs. Physicians are salaried or they bill separately for their professional fees.

Hospital associated. The hospital governs and manages the ambulatory-care program, which is financed through a contractual arrangement of shared expenses and revenue with physicians.

Hospital as landlord. The hospital provides or leases space in which physicians locate their office practices, but the physicians assume total fiscal accountability for their ambulatory-care practices.

Another set of terms is necessary for describing the location of the facility:

Hospital based. The facility is located on the main hospital campus.

Satellite. The facility is located off the hospital campus.

Two meanings and interpretations are ascribed to the freestanding ambulatory-care center. To some health-industry observers, *freestanding* refers to a facility that is physically separate from any other health facility. This interpretation does not address the presence or absence of organizational linkage. In this interpretation of the term, hospitals as well as other providers of health services, can sponsor or manage a freestanding ambulatory-care center. This chapter will use this interpretation throughout the following discussion.

In the second interpretation of the term, *freestanding* means both a physically separate facility and a facility and program corporately and legally distinct from any other organization. In this sense, by definition, all freestanding ambulatory-care centers are physically separate and organizationally distinct from hospitals.

In summary, a *freestanding ambulatory-care center* connotes a facility physically separate from another health facility. However, the freestanding ambulatory-care center may vary according to governance structures, types of ownership and sponsorship, comprehensiveness of services, and types of affiliation with hospitals.

A hospital's involvement in or control of an ambulatory-care program can vary with the type of ambulatory service. For example, a hospital might control all aspects of a primary-care group practice, including payment of physicians' salaries, while being involved only as a building landlord for a facility in which private-practice physicians offer subspecialized services. Table 7–1 displays an analysis of a hypothetical hospital's involvement in ambulatory care.

Reasons for Hospital Involvement in Ambulatory Care

It is essential for policymakers to understand the factors motivating hospitals to establish or expand their ambulatory-care programs. Various motiva-

Table 7–1
Matrix of Hospital Ambulatory-Care Programs

	Type of Ambulatory Program		
Degree of Hospital Control	*Program I: Ambulatory Surgery*	*Program II: Interdisciplinary Pain Program*	*Program III: General Medical Program*
Ownership of facility	Hospital	Hospital	Hospital
Administrative services such as billing	Hospital	Hospital	Hospital
Shared services: purchasing, laundry	Hospital	Hospital	Hospital
Management	Hospital	Hospital	Private medical group
Supervision and compensation allied health personnel	Hospital	Hospital	Private medical group
Operating subsidy	Hospital	Hospital	Hospital/group
Capital financing	Hospital	Hospital	Hospital
Physician compensation	Surgeons bill separately for professional service	Physicians bill separately	Private medical group

Source: Reprinted from Linda A. Burns, "Will Multi-Institutional Systems Serve as Change Agents to Improve the Management of Ambulatory Care?" *Journal of Ambulatory Care Management* 3 (August 1980): 6. By permission of Aspen Systems Corporation, copyright 1980.

tions can be ascribed to hospitals that develop or expand ambulatory care; these have been discussed elsewhere.[3] In addition to technological changes, other motivating influences can be identified such as changing demand for health services; shifting preferences of third-party payers and regulators; feeder for inpatient programs; diversification of risk; competitive influences; economies of scale; economies of scope; mission statement of hospital; teaching programs; and research programs.

Hospital Legal Structures

Besides understanding various hospital roles and motivations in operating various ambulatory services, decision makers should recognize a fundamental change that is occurring in the legal structures of hospitals. This change in legal structures has not been reflected in hospital-industry data bases, and thus the extent to which hospitals provide ambulatory care may be understated. Historically, hospitals, especially nonprofit institutions, have not concerned themselves greatly with legal structure. However, dramatic changes in their operating environments have made it essential for hospitals to protect existing assets and income and to increase net revenues. Increased net revenues are necessary to replace fixed assets, meet the growing demand from the aging population, finance unreimbursed care, and finance technological improvements. As a result of these pressures, the traditional hospital corporate structure is increasingly being replaced by a corporate structure consisting of a parent holding company with subsidiary companies, only one of which may "produce" acute inpatient care. The other subsidiaries might produce ambulatory care, home care, and long-term care, as well as manage nonhealth enterprises.

Cost comparisons among ambulatory-care providers should take into account these new corporate legal structures. Aggregate hospital-industry statistics conceal the wide variation in organizational arrangements that hospitals and physicians use to provide ambulatory care. While the organized OPD staffed with salaried physicians is the arrangement one typically thinks of, in fact, there is a large and growing variety of ways in which hospitals and physicians cooperate to provide such care. For example, increasing numbers of hospitals are reorganizing their ambulatory-care programs so that the ambulatory services are financed and managed according to the terms of a contractual arrangement with physicians. These physicians typically are not employees of the hospital but do share financial risks and gains incurred through the operation of ambulatory care within the hospital. The costs of operating the ambulatory-care programs are recovered through a variety of billing arrangements: (1) The hospital bills third-party payers and/or patients for both physician- and hospital-incurred costs;

(2) the physician bills third-party payers or patients for both physician-
and hospital-incurred costs; and (3) the hospital bills for its costs and the
physicians bill for their costs, in effect, rendering two bills for distinct
components of the total costs of operating the ambulatory-care program. In
other cases, hospitals are segregating their ambulatory-care services into
corporations that are legally and organizationally distinct from the hospital
corporation as discussed earlier.

Hospitals with organized ambulatory-care programs vary by size of
hospital, type of control, and teaching status. Ambulatory-care programs
managed by hospitals also vary in organizational structure and financial
relationships with physicians.

Hospitals with organized ambulatory-care programs tend to be larger
than the average-sized hospitals. Of all hospitals, 49 percent have OPDs; 80
percent of hospitals with 400–499 beds have OPDs; and 82 percent of all
hospitals with more than 500 beds have OPDs, as shown in table 7–2.[4] In
1980, 70 percent of all hospitals with OPDs were private, nonprofit, and
another 21 percent of such hospitals were government, nonfederal hospitals.
Private, investor-owned hospitals account for only 9 percent of the total
number of hospitals with OPDs, as shown in table 7–3. While teaching

Table 7–2
Community Hospitals with Outpatient Departments,
by Bed Size, 1980

Bed Size	All Hospitals	Hospitals with OPDs	Percent with OPDs
Under 100	2,838	733	25.8
100–199	1,379	656	47.6
200–299	716	454	63.4
300–399	413	315	76.3
400–499	267	213	79.8
500 or over	317	260	82.0
Totals	5,916	2,631	44.5

Source: American Hospital Association 1980 Annual Survey.

Table 7–3
Number and Percent of Community Hospitals with Outpatient
Departments by Type of Control, 1980

Hospital Control	Total	Number with OPDs	Percent of All Hospitals with OPDs	Percent of Hospitals with Same Control
Government nonfederal	1,803	551	21	31
Private, nonprofit	3,349	1,841	70	55
Private, investor owned	764	239	9	31
Totals	5,916	2,631	100	

Source: American Hospital Association 1980 Annual Survey.

hospitals account for 29 percent of hospitals with OPDs, teaching hospitals with OPDs account for 64 percent of all OPD visits. The average size of an OPD in a teaching hospital is 76,043 annual visits contrasted with the average size of an OPD in a nonteaching hospital of 17,460 annual visits, as depicted in table 7–4.

These aggregate statistics mask some significant distributional aspects of ambulatory care. The poor, the uneducated, and the nonwhite population use OPDs and EDs more frequently than the rest of the population. There is likely to be a close relationship between beneficiaries of the Medicaid program and those who use OPDs.

Costs and the Hospital OPD

A significant unresolved issue is determining the cost of ambulatory care provided by hospitals. The proper measure of cost for public or private decision making is marginal cost. Currently the estimates of costs of hospital ambulatory care are based on accounting techniques that usually provide a measure of average cost. They allocate a significant portion of the hospital's overhead cost to the ambulatory-care programs by using a methodology that is both arbitrary and misleading for decision-making purposes. For example, part of the cost of operating a twenty-four hour laboratory might be assigned to the OPD. But it can be argued that this is not a true cost to the OPD since the hospital would operate the laboratory for the same hours even in the absence of the OPD. Typically more than half of a hospital's total costs are allocated as overhead,[6] so the margin of error in the amount of costs allocated to ambulatory care is quite substantial.

At present, estimates of the cost of outpatient care come from accounting records and usually consist of two parts. First, total direct costs incurred by accounts charged to the department in question are counted. Next, some part of the hospital's overhead costs—those costs that are not charged to any specific output—are allocated to the department. The method of allocation is usually some kind of step-down procedure, based on fairly arbitrary indicators of relative volume such as square footage, share of direct costs, or counts of services. The sum of average direct and indirect or overhead costs divided by total visits or units of service is then called the "cost of unit of ambulatory care." Such estimates have been obtained for New York City hospitals,[7,8] eight hospitals in the Northeast and Midwest,[9] one hospital in Indianapolis,[10] and the radiology department of one hypothetical hospital.[11]

These procedures and the studies that used them are subject to several objections. First, only small samples or a single hospital have been investigated; no large-sample, much less a nationwide, estimate of the cost of hospital ambulatory care exists. Second, the actual estimates of cost depend a great deal on the basis used for allocating overhead cost. Olmstead, for

Table 7-4
Number and Percent of Community Hospitals with Outpatient
Departments by Teaching Status, 1980

Hospital characteristics	Teaching	Nonteaching	Total
Total number of hospitals	970	4,946	5,916
Number with OPD	765	1,866	2,631
Percent of hospitals with OPD	79	38	44
Number of OPD visits (in millions)	58,173	32,580	90,753
Percent of all visits	64	36	100
Average visits per hospital OPD	76,043	17,460	34,494

Source: American Hospital Association 1980 Annual Survey

example, found large shifts in estimates of relative housekeeping costs for inpatient and outpatient care depending on whether square footage or hours of service were used for allocation. Third, the use of time-motion or other intensive and detailed methods to allocate overhead costs is itself costly, time-consuming, and controversial. A method that could avoid these problems would be highly valued. Finally, and most fundamentally, these procedures are arbitrary. They are arbitrary in the obvious sense that the cost estimates will differ depending on what basis is used to allocate overhead costs. They are also arbitrary in the important sense that there is no ideal basis for allocating those costs. It is not just a question of which approximation to an ideal is to be used but rather that there is no ideal.

A project currently underway at the American Hospital Association, with funding from the Health Care Financing Administration is attempting to facilitate the analysis of hospital OPD costs. The project will generate a data base on the extent and costs of ambulatory care provided by hospitals. In addition, the data is expected to provide a baseline for monitoring the growth of hospital-sponsored and associated ambulatory care. The data base, when complete, should provide a rich and varied resource for policy analysis.

One area for exploration in this project will be marginal costs of providing outpatient services. The data collected in the study will permit estimation of marginal costs using flexible-form, multiproduct-cost functions. This method has been developed extensively by econometricians in recent years, and it has been applied to hospitals but not with emphasis on ambulatory care.

The multiproduct-cost function provides a somewhat less arbitrary procedure for allocating these costs, using data for a sample of hospitals on total hospital costs, levels of inpatient and outpatient services provided, prices of inputs, and other factors that might influence costs. In this approach, econometric procedures (typically regression models of some type) are used to estimate a mathematical relationship between total hospital costs and the mix and levels of inpatient and outpatient care, while controlling for differences across hospitals in input prices and other factors that may influence costs. The estimated relationship can then be used to predict the cost of providing a given level of inpatient and outpatient care for a hospital facing a given set of prices and operating in a given environment (defined by factors such as the type and complexity of cases served, whether the hospital is for-profit or not, and hospital location).

The cost function can also be used to derive estimates of the "marginal" costs of inpatient and outpatient care, that is, the cost of serving one additional outpatient or providing one additional inpatient day of care, for hospitals with given characteristics. The estimated-cost function will yield marginal costs that vary with the current levels of services (reflecting economies or diseconomies of scale) if such a relationship between costs and service levels is uncovered in the econometric estimation. A wide variety of interesting results pertaining to hospital costs and efficiency can be derived from the estimated multiproduct-cost function.

The importance of this issue of cost of hospital ambulatory care can be emphasized by recognizing the multiple roles that hospital ambulatory-care programs play in the overall medical-care system. On the one hand, they are envisioned as less costly substitutes for inpatient care, as in the case of ambulatory surgery that might substitute for inpatient surgery. On the other hand, OPDs and EDs substitute for the services of private physicians' offices, and the relevant question is the relative cost of the alternatives. Since many patients, particularly Medicare and Medicaid beneficiaries, have no price incentives to choose the least costly alternative (even if the prices accurately reflect costs), the likelihood of choosing the least costly source of care is fairly low. It seems most likely, and has been shown,[12] that when money prices are zero, time and convenience costs become the dominant force in selecting providers. As Medicaid fees are lowered, private physicians become less willing to accept Medicaid patients,[13] and, so it is argued, Medicaid patients react to the reduced availability of private physicians and seek ambulatory care at hospitals. Similarly, Medicare patients may be more likely to use hospital ambulatory-care programs if there are not enough physicians willing to accept assignment of Medicare. Whether the resource or program cost at an OPD or ED is greater or less than at the private physician's office is irrelevant to the patients since they do not face a money price. But the resource costs of the alternatives are real, as are program costs borne by the taxpayer. A major goal of this project is to estimate the marginal resource cost of the various types of hospital-provided ambulatory services.

Institutional Effects on the Cost of Care

At least three issues related to the organizational arrangement of hospital ambulatory-care programs are likely to affect the cost of care and relate to the policy choices of interest to both the industry and third-party payers, including the government. The issues are economies of scale (that is, whether or not costs per unit of service decline as the size of the OPD increases); of economies of scope (that is, whether ambulatory services are produced more cheaply in combination with other hospital services or in separate physician offices); and the effect of physician financial incentives on cost. For example, a recently completed study of medical group practices shows:

> Decreasing returns to scale, that is, cost per unit of output *increase* as the size of the medical group *increases*, although the rate of cost increase was quantitatively quite small.

> A dramatic and quantitatively large effect of the financial incentives confronting the group's physicians on economic efficiency, that is, to the effect that the closer a physician's own financial welfare is affected by his or her own performance, the more productive is the physician.[14]

Since the study looked only at office-based practices, it could not deal with the issue of economies of scope. These three issues are important to understanding the issue of the cost of ambulatory care provided in hospitals, and the issues relate to the type and size of OPDs and EDs that should or should not be encouraged. This information will be useful to both the hospital industry and third-party payers, including the government.

Unique Market Aspects of Hospital Ambulatory Care

To understand the cost of care provided in OPDs and EDs, policymakers must also consider the issue of what markets OPDs serve. If some OPDs serve markets that other providers such as private physicians' offices could not serve at the same total real cost, then policy choices will need to consider the alternatives open to society. For example, some OPDs may serve inner-city markets where competing forms of ambulatory care may not be available at the same time or convenience cost. If convenient accessibility to medical care for everyone continues to be a major social goal, then the total cost of alternatives to the OPD will need to be taken into account.

Conclusion

Hospitals provide a large portion of the total ambulatory care relied on in the United States. Clinical services provided by hospitals on an ambulatory basis include both primary care and high-technology and subspecialty services. There are a growing variety of types of organizational arrangements hospitals use to provide ambulatory care, and few data exist today that accurately or completely describe hospital ambulatory-care programs. Thus discussions about the relative costs of hospital ambulatory care compared to other providers are hindered by lack of data.

Notes

1. American Hospital Association, *Hospital Statistics* (Chicago: American Hospital Association, 1981), p. 186.
2. L.A. Burns and M. Ferber, "Definitions Proposed for Hospital Roles in Ambulatory Care," *Outreach* (July/August 1980): 3, American Hospital Association.
3. L.A. Burns, "Will Multi-Institutional Systems Serve as Change Agents to Improve the Management of Ambulatory Care?" *Journal of Ambulatory Care Management* 3 (1980): Vol. 3, no. 3 1–17.
4. American Hospital Association Annual Survey, 1980.
5. See T. Lowing and A.G. Hollmann and Roddy (1980).
6. Jeffrey Harris, "Pricing Rules for Hospitals," *Bell Journal of Economics* 10 (Spring 1979): 224–243.
7. Greater New York Hospital Association, "Ambulatory Care: An Overview and Comparative Analysis of Hospital-Based and Freestanding Delivery Systems," unpublished manuscript, June 1979.
8. D. Epple and U. Reinhardt, "Analysis of the Cost of Ambulatory Care at New York City Hospitals," unpublished manuscript, 1971.
9. F. Olmstead, *Final Report and Analysis and Evaluative Methodologies for Determining Ambulatory Care Costs* (Silver Spring, Md.: Orkand Corporation, 1979).
10. S. Roberts, "Cost Analysis of Outpatient Care and Its Implica-

tions," in *Improving Ambulatory Health Delivery*, ed. G. Lasdon (Lexington, Mass.: D.C. Heath/LexingtonBooks, 1976), pp. 113–134.

11. J.D. Glavas, "Outpatient Treatment a Good Way to Reduce Hospital Costs," *Hospital Financial Management* 4 (June 1974).

12. See, for example, Jay Helms, Joseph P. Newhouse, and Charles E. Phelps, "Copayments and Demand for Medical Care: The California Medicaid Experience," *Bell Journal of Economics* 9 (Spring 1978): 192–208.

13. See, for example, Jack Hadley, "Physician Participation in Medicaid, Evidence from California," Urban Institute Paper 998–18 (Washington, D.C., January 1979); Frank A. Sloan, Jerry Cromwell, and Janet B. Mitchell, *Private Physicians and Public Programs* (Lexington, Mass.: D.C. Heath/LexingtonBooks, 1978); and Philip J. Held, Larry Manheim, and Judith Wooldridge, "Physician Acceptance of Medicaid Patients," unpublished paper. (Princeton, N.J.: Mathematica Policy Research) 1978.

14. Philip J. Held and Uwe Reinhardt, eds., *An Analysis of Economic Performance of Medical Group Practices* (Princeton, N.J.: Mathematica Policy Research, 9, 1979).

8

Hospital-Sponsored Primary-Care Group Practice: Preliminary Findings from a National Evaluation

Thomas M. Wickizer and
Stephen M. Shortell

The role of community hospitals in ambulatory care is changing significantly. Among the more important factors that have led hospitals to reevaluate their approaches to providing ambulatory care have been: the dramatic growth in the demand for hospital outpatient care,[1,2] the need to increase the efficiency of hospital outpatient services,[3] quality-of-care considerations,[4,5] and the changing nature of the market for hospital services.[6,7] These factors have led to efforts to initiate change and to extend the hospital's role in ambulatory care beyond traditional emergency-room services and outpatient-clinic arrangements. Among the organizational initiatives being developed by hospitals are expansion of hospital primary-care facilities, development of satellite clinics for primary care, participation in health-maintenance organization (HMO) activity, and development of ambulatory-surgery units.[8,9]

One initiative that has received particular interest and attention is the development of hospital-sponsored, primary-care group practice.[10–12] Although reports of the experience of individual hospitals in starting group practices have appeared in the literature,[13–15] systematic study of this innovation has so far been limited. This chapter presents some preliminary findings from an evaluation of a national demonstration program involving hospitals that have attempted to initiate change in the area of ambulatory care through the development of primary-care group practice.

The Demonstration Program

Approximately seven years ago the Robert Wood Johnson Foundation (RWJF) mounted a national demonstration program, the Community Hospital Program (CHP), formerly called the Community Hospital/Medical Staff Sponsored Primary Care Group Practice Program. The purpose of the CHP was to improve access to general medical care and to as-

The research reported here was supported by grants from the Robert Wood Johnson Foundation, Princeton, New Jersey.

sist community hospitals in strengthening their role in ambulatory care through the development of hospital-sponsored, primary-care group practice (HSPCGP).[16,17] All nonprofit, short-term general hospitals were eligible to participate in the demonstration program, with the exception of hospitals with major teaching involvement. Of approximately 900 hospitals that were invited to participate in the program, 225 submitted applications, and 54 of these accepted grants of up to $500,000 originally for a period not to exceed four years (although many received a one-year grant extension). The grant awards were made over a three-year period beginning in 1976 (at present eleven of the fifty-three grantees are active in the CHP and continue to receive funding). Prior experience with ambulatory care or the existence of clinics or other outpatient services were not in themselves determinants of eligibility for funding. To assure geographic distribution of programs, there were initial limitations on the number of hospitals in any one state that could be funded.

The grants were to be used for program planning and development and to offset operating deficits during the start-up phase of operation. Physicians hired to staff the group practices were to be employees of the hospital or, singly or as a group, could enter into professional service contracts with the hospital to provide patient care. Administrative- and medical-support staff of the groups were to be hospital employees. Finally, the groups were expected to continue to operate under hospital sponsorship after the end of the grant period.

Placing group practices under hospital/medical-staff sponsorship was believed to have several benefits: to improve the hospitals' role in delivering primary care; to provide better integration of primary care with secondary and tertiary care; to promote continuity of care; and to enable the group practice to capitalize on the back-up support capabilities of the hospital including laboratory, x-ray, social work, physical therapy, home health care, patient education, and related services. From the patient's viewpoint it was felt that this arrangement would result in a number of advantages including availability of a personal physician with back-up support; a central medical-record system; provision of twenty-four-hour medical care, thereby eliminating the need to rely solely on the hospital emergency room; establishment of a group of physicians and staff in a single setting to provide continuous care for the entire family; and organization of a referral system to coordinate primary care and specialty care.

The Evaluation: Questions and Study Design

In order to learn as much as possible from this major demonstration program, the Robert Wood Johnson Foundation has funded an evaluation being conducted by the University of Washington Department of Health Services.

This evaluation is focused on three major questions:

1. To what degree does the program strengthen the hospitals' ongoing commitment to providing organized primary-care services to their communities? In so doing, to what degree is the *organization* of access to primary-care services improved?
2. To what degree does the program strengthen the financial viability of the sponsoring hospital in terms of the impact on admissions, market share of admissions, ancillary-services use, and referrals to staff specialists?
3. To what degree does the program result in financially viable, primary-care group practices?

Because of the complexity and nature of the demonstration program, the evaluation has employed a distinctly "triangulated"[18] approach to address the preceding questions. This design, described in detail elsewhere,[19] has involved a combination of single-time-series design and longitudinal comparative case studies using a variety of primary and secondary data-collection sources. The single-time-series design has involved the collection of quantitative data on all fifty-three grantees at various times during the grant-funding period. Data have also been collected on grantees prior to funding and during a specified follow-up period after funding. The data are being analyzed through multivariate techniques to assess the factors associated with the different performance outcomes of the groups.

The second component of the evaluation involves the collection of qualitative data through longitudinal comparative case studies being conducted in thirteen of the fifty-three sites. Twelve case-study sites from among thirty-six grantees funded as of July 1, 1977, were selected for analysis based on stratified random sampling. A thirteenth case-study site was subsequently added at its request because of geographical convenience to the evaluation team. The case-study grantees are similar to grantees at large in most respects except they are larger and have more outpatient visits.

The thirteen case-study sites have been visited by two study-team members once each year since receiving the grant award. A detailed semistructured questionnaire protocol is used to interview a number of individuals associated with the practice, including hospital administrators, governing-board members, selected hospital medical-staff members, group managers, group medical directors, and group physicians. Virtually every aspect of the group's formation, organization, and operations is covered in the comprehensive interviews. The interviews are recorded and transcribed, and then summaries are developed containing all the substantive information obtained. A more detailed description of the sample-selection processs and case-study protocol is provided elsewhere.[20]

To document the performance of grantees involved in the CHP, measures and criteria related to the three major questions being addressed by the evaluation have been developed. Given the multiple objectives of the program, however, it seems oversimplified and misleading to characterize a grantee's experience as a success or failure. A more useful approach is to think of the various dimensions in terms of constituting a *performance profile*. It is the rare grantee that will score consistently high or consistently low on all the many dimensions. Rather, it is expected that most grantees will score high on some dimensions and not so high on others. By taking a more refined, performance-profile approach, it becomes possible not only to make fine-grained distinctions regarding outcomes but, most important, to understand *why* groups did so well on some dimensions and not so well on others. For example, the factors associated with strengthening the hospitals' role on some dimensions may have impeded their achievement of others. Similarly, the factors that may be associated with a fiscally viable group practice may not be the same factors associated with an overall stronger role for the hospital in primary care.

A behavioral model has been developed to provide a framework for considering those factors likely to be associated with different performance criteria. The external demand-and-supply factors and hospital-specific characteristics are expected to influence the program-design and management factors, which in turn are expected to influence provider productivity and turnover. The performance-profile indicators involving the hospitals' strengthened role in primary care, the contribution of a group to the hospitals' fiscal health, and a group's own financial viability are each expected to be a function of provider productivity and turnover, the program design and management factors, and the demand, supply, and hospital-specific factors. The basic thesis of this model that guides the evaluation is that how well a group does on the performance profile will largely be associated with how well it is designed and managed (that is, the strategic choices and methods of implementing the program), taking into account community demand-and-supply factors and hospital-specific variables.

The Study Hospitals

Because data on all fifty-three sites in the CHP are still in the process of being collected and analyzed, the data reported here are restricted to the thirteen sites selected for case-study analysis. Since these sites were funded and began operation earlier in the demonstration program, they provide a sample for which reasonably complete data can be reported. As noted previously, the case-study sites are representative of the first thirty-six sites that were funded in the demonstration program. Furthermore, they do not differ significantly on a number of characteristics from the seventeen sites that were later funded, although they do tend to be larger, located in nonrural areas, and have more previous primary-care experience. Table 8–1 summarizes selected characteristics of the thirteen sites.

As shown, the hospitals range in bed size from 78 to 697 beds, with an average bed size of 386. This compares to 165 beds for community hospitals at large. As could be expected, given their comparatively large size, the study hospitals have more admissions and outpatient visits than community hospitals overall. On the average, the study hospitals had 10,997 admissions and 89,694 outpatient visits during 1977 (the relatively high average number of outpatient visits of the study hospitals is due in part to the very high number of visits reported by one hospital) compared to 5,827 admissions and 33,780 outpatient visits for community hospitals nationwide, as reported by the American Hospital Association. With respect to occupancy rate, the study hospitals appear to be quite similar to community hospitals overall.

Although the hospitals differed in a number of respects, they shared the common characteristic of being located, for the most part, in underserved communities, which included both urban and rural areas as well as various geographical regions. Four of the hospitals were located in low-income urban areas where the estimated primary-care physician-to-population ratio was approximately 0.35/1,000 to 0.70/1,000. Four other hospitals were located in rural areas that had experienced long-standing problems in recruiting primary-care physicians. In one of the communities the primary-care physician-to-population ratio was estimated to be 0.25/1,000, and about one-third of the population reported having no regular source of care.

In regard to the groups themselves, table 8–1 reveals that seven of the thirteen are multispecialty groups, located primarily in urban areas. Only five of the thirteen started completely from scratch in building a practice. Of the remaining eight, three were preexisting practices (at least in part), and the others represented reorganized OPD efforts and/or situations in which at least one of the physicians in practice in the community brought in patients to the new primary-care group practice. Seven of the thirteen sites used nurse practitioners or physician assistants (five using nurse practitioners and two using physician assistants). Eight of the thirteen sites were located off hospital grounds, and three operated several delivery sites.

Preliminary Findings

The preliminary findings presented in the following discussion and in tables 8–2 through 8–7 consist of descriptive data on selected performance mea-

Table 8–1
Selected Characteristics of Case-Study Hospitals and Groups

Hospital	Out-patient Visits	Total Beds[a]	Admissions[a]	Occupancy[a] (Percent)	Hospitals' Experience in Primary Care	Hospital Location	Multi- or Single-Specialty	Preexisting Site, Reorganized OPD, or Doctor Brought in Patients	Use Nurse Practitioners or Physician Assistants	On/Off Hospital Grounds	More than One Site
A	101,981	530	18,117	82.5	High	Urban	Multispecialty	In part, reorganized OPD	No	Off	No
B	133,716	328	11,511	83.8	High	Urban	Multispecialty	Preexisting	Yes	Off	No
C[b]	95,586	185	7,529	51.5	None	Rural	Single specialty (family practice)	No	No	Off	No
D	478,954	697	23,258	88.8	High	Suburban	Multispecialty	Preexisting in part and doctors brought in patients	Yes	On	No
E	82,513	406	13,742	87.1	Some	Urban	Multispecialty	Preexisting site, in part	Yes	Both	Yes
F	63,820	556	18,009	73.5	Some	Urban	Single specialty (family practice)	No	Yes	Off	No
G	22,402	78	2,911	73.1	None	Rural	Single specialty (family practice)	No	Yes	Off	No
H	27,074	342	12,487	71.1	Some	Urban	Single specialty (family practice)	One doctor brought in patients	No	Off	No
I	62,349	259	11,061	73.4	Some	Suburban	Multispecialty	Preexisting site	No	Off	Yes
J	74,238	191	7,646	76.1	Some	Rural	Single specialty (family practice)	No	Yes	Off	Yes
K	36,447	194	6,209	80.4	Some	Urban	Multispecialty	Reorganized OPD and doctors brought in patients	Yes	On	No
L	56,553	389	12,247	63.2	None	Urban	Multispecialty	Reorganized OPD in part	No	On	No
M	21,078	251	9,240	76.9	High	Urban	Single specialty (family practice)	No	No	On	No

[a]Based on data collected by the American Hospital Association 1977 Annual Survey.

[b]This site represents two hospitals that are jointly sponsoring the project. Data for this site reflect the combined totals for the separate hospitals, except for occupancy, which is an averaged value.

sures. The data are reported by site for each study hospital as well as for the hospitals overall. It should be emphasized that the information presented here represents preliminary findings based on a limited number of cases. Considerable caution should therefore be used in interpreting the information. More complete findings and more detailed analysis from the evaluation of the CHP will be presented in future reports.[21]

Impact on the Hospital's Commitment to Provide
Primary Care and on the Organization of Access to Care

One of the principal questions being addressed by the evaluation concerns whether hospitals involved in the CHP develop a continuing commitment to provide primary ambulatory care. One way to answer this question is to examine the degree to which the groups or the sponsoring hospitals themselves continue to offer innovative services over the period of the grant. For sites for which data exist for both the baseline and the time at which the group went off the grant, the data suggest that there has been a greater percentage growth in the number of organized innovative services offered by the group practice (120 percent) and innovative services offered by the hospital (42 percent and 85 percent) than the relative percentage increase in services offered by community organizations (38 percent and 21 percent). These data, while preliminary, suggest that the demonstration program has had some effect on stimulating the further development of organized primary-care efforts on the part of hospitals in their communities.

A related question concerns the degree to which the *organization* of access to primary-care services improves as a result of the hospitals' involvement in the demonstration program. One way of addressing this question is to examine the impact of the groups on hospital ER services. It was the intent that the primary-care groups would provide a better alternative for the treatment of nonurgent patients seeking care from hospital ERs and for patients without a personal physician to provide needed follow-up care. Although the percentage of visits to the groups resulting from referrals of patients from the hospital ER has overall remained quite small, the data indicate there has been some increase over time in referrals of both nonurgent patients and patients needing follow-up care. For groups that have gone off the grant for which data are available, approximately 7 percent of patient visits were estimated to result from the referral of nonurgent patients and the referral of patients for follow-up care during the operational period prior to the end of grant funding.

To the extent that the groups are having a positive effect on the organization of access to care, one would hope to see an increase over time in the percentage of patients classified as "urgent" treated in the hospital ER, with nonurgent patients and patients without a physician needing follow-up care being referred to the primary-care group. Data are available through year 3 of operation for most of the case-study sites. From year 1 to year 3 of operation, the data indicate that the percentage of ER visits classified as urgent increased by slightly over 4 percent. Although preliminary, the data suggest that primary-care groups sponsored by hospitals can have some impact on improving the organization of access to general medical-care services.

Effects on the Sponsoring Hospital

The second principal question being addressed concerns the degree to which the program strengthened the financial viability of the sponsoring hospital in terms of impact on admissions, ancillary-services use, improving the hospital's market share for inpatient services, and related measures. This question is especially important to hospital administrators and others who may be involved in the planning of HSPCGPs. Although hospitals considering sponsorship of a primary-care group practice are motivated by the desire to serve their·communities, they must also be concerned with meeting their own institutional goals. Further, because a hospital-sponsored group's revenues may not be sufficient to cover its costs even in the long run, hospitals must consider the possibility that continued subsidization of the group may be necessary. A hospital's willingness to subsidize its group over a long period of time depends in part on the benefits it accrues from that subsidization program.

Table 8–2 summarizes the percentage of hospital admissions accounted for by group patients by year of operation. There appears to be some increase in the percentage of hospital admissions accounted for by group patients over time, although this is not a consistent pattern across all sites. Most groups for which data are available account for between 2 and 4 percent of total hospital inpatient admissions. However, this does not include admissions of patients, referred to specialists, who may subsequently be hospitalized. Groups overall have reported that approximately 7 percent of patient visits result in referral to hospital specialist staff. Hence, the data reported in table 8–2 underestimate the actual effect of groups on hospital inpatient admissions. While it appears that most of the groups have had a limited effect on the hospital in terms of direct admissions, at least one site (hospital E) stands out. This group, which is a multispecialty practice with satellite sites in addition to a hospital-based site, accounted for nearly 10 percent of total hospital admissions through direct admissions of patients by the fourth operational year.

Table 8–2
Percentage of Hospital Admissions Accounted for by Group Patients,
by Year of Group Operation

Hospital	Year 1 of Operation (N = 10) (Percent)	Year 2 of Operation (N = 13) (Percent)	Year 3 of Operation (N = 12) (Percent)	Year 4 of Operation (N = 6) (Percent)
A	0.30	0.42	3.20	b
B	0.20	1.80	2.00	1.52
C	0.90	6.51	3.30	b
D	1.30	1.93	1.20	b
E	4.50	7.78	7.40	9.50
F	0.30	4.55	2.40	2.60
G	1.50	2.36	0.90	1.00
H	a	1.28	2.30	6.21
I	a	3.35	b	b
J	a	0.78	0.00	b
K	4.20	3.96	3.70	b
L	<0.01	<0.01	<0.01	b
M	0.30	0.60	1.00	0.43
Mean	1.32	2.72	2.28	3.54
S.D.	1.68	2.41	2.03	3.57
Range	0.01–4.50	0.01–7.78	0–7.40	0.43–9.50

[a]Data not reported for this year.
[b]Data not available because hospital went off grant prior to completing operational period.

A second area where primary-care groups may affect the hospital is in use of ancillary services. Table 8–3 summarizes the volume of hospital laboratory tests and x-ray exams generated by groups by year of operation. What is not known is what proportion of total hospital ancillary revenue this represents. Information obtained through the case studies, however, suggests that with few exceptions this is less than 10 percent and usually closer to 2 to 5 percent. To a large extent, the volume of ancillary services generated by hospital-sponsored groups depends on the practice location. Groups located on hospital grounds usually use the hospital's laboratory and x-ray more frequently and thus generate a greater volume of hospital ancillary services. Compared to satellite sites, groups located on the hospital grounds generated approximately twice the volume of hospital laboratory tests and three times the volume of hospital x-ray exams.

The limited information presented here suggests that primary-care groups can have an effect on hospitals in terms of use of inpatient and ancillary services. One important question not addressed is whether the development of a primary-care group can also affect the hospital's market share relative to its competitors. Data pertaining to this question are currently being examined, with preliminary results suggesting that HSPCGPs can increase the hospital's market share.[22]

Table 8-3
Volume of Hospital Laboratory Tests and X-Ray Exams Generated,
by Group by Year of Operation

	Year 2 of Operation		Year 3 of Operation		Year 4 of Operation	
Hospital	*Lab Tests* *(N = 12)*	*X-Ray Exams* *(N = 11)*	*Lab Tests* *(N = 12)*	*X-Ray Exams* *(N = 12)*	*Lab Tests* *(N = 6)*	*X-Ray Exams* *(N = 6)*
A	3,565	360	7,260	520	b	b
B	a	a	11,932	1,627	10,560	1,440
C	1,170	900	2,051	1,034	b	b
D	6,062	390	15,600	1,972	b	b
E	5,656	1,342	8,222	2,026	9,780	1,833
F	537	a	335	250	458	260
G	394	100	740	85	792	100
H	0	36	0	50	0	65
I	1,913	0	b	b	b	b
J	480	275	1,500	0	b	b
K	1,504	543	2,000	614	b	b
L	5,800	978	6,034	1,207	b	b
M	32	210	50	432	43	429
Mean	2,259	467	4,643	818	3,605	687
S.D.	2,370	433	5,176	741	5,099	756
Range	0–6,062	0–1,342	0–15,600	0–2,026	0–10,560	65–1,833

Note: Where necessary the data have been adjusted to reflect twelve-month periods of operation.

[a]Data not reported for this year.

[b]Data not reported because hospital went off grant prior to completing operational period.

Group Financial Viability

The third major question being addressed by the evaluation concerns whether hospital-sponsored groups achieve financial viability. Tables 8-4 through 8-6 present data on three different measures related to group financial viability. Table 8-4 summarizes data on direct cost per visit, inflation adjusted to reflect January 1980 prices. As shown, the average cost per visit declines over time, reflecting increased efficiency of operations. The average cost per visit during the third-year operational period (the last period of operation for which data for most groups are available) is $31.48. The five groups for which data are available for the fourth-year operational period had an average cost per visit of $26.61. Because of differences in cost-accounting procedures and the lack of uniformity in measurement, it is difficult to make precise comparisons across settings with regard to costs. In general, however, the costs of HSPCGP reported here compare very favorably with those reported for other settings including private physicians' offices.[23-27]

Table 8-5 summarizes data pertaining to the number of visits per

Table 8–4
Cost per Visit, by Months of Operation
(dollars)

Hospital	Number of Months of Operation			
	1–12 *(n = 13)*	*13–24* *(n = 13)*	*24–36* *(n = 11)*	*37–48* *(n = 5)*
A	58.75	62.23	29.72	a
B	52.55	31.41	23.02	24.24
C	81.24	34.33	b	b
D	75.11	69.60	34.87	a
E	31.24	25.41	25.58	21.24
F	53.71	24.12	26.75	27.90
G	49.83	40.76	30.81	24.98
H	78.54	51.63	34.00	b
I	34.48	35.41	a	a
J	36.18	40.29	25.34	a
K	87.13	38.49	26.34	a
L	72.00	41.28	40.72	a
M	227.40	199.91	49.17	34.70
Mean	72.17	53.45	31.48	26.61
S.D.	50.20	45.93	7.82	5.10
Range	31.24–227.40	24.12–199.91	23.02–49.17	21.24–34.70

Note: Costs include only *direct operating expenses*. Data adjusted by the monthly CPI to reflect January 1980 prices.
[a]Data not available because hospital went off grant prior to completing operational period.
[b]Data not yet available for groups due to the length of time in operation.

full-time equivalent (FTE) physician by months of operation. As shown, the average number of visits per FTE physician increased from 2,300 in the first twelve-month operational period to 4,073 during the fourth-year period. Given that these groups represent newly established developing practices, these findings are noteworthy. Of the five groups for which data are available for the fourth operational year, two had a level of productivity near or above that reported for *established* family-practice groups nationwide according to unpublished data from the Medical Group Management Association.

Finally, table 8–6 presents data on operating margin, a key indicator of financial viability, that provides a measure of revenues in relation to direct costs. As shown, the operating margin for groups decreases from −0.623 during the first twelve-month operational period to −0.230 during the fourth-year operational period, reflecting a favorable growth in revenues relative to costs and greater efficiency of group operations. As table 8–6 shows, two groups (sites E and M) operated very near the point of break-even (based on direct costs and net operating revenues) during the fourth-year period.

Table 8-5
Visits per Full-Time Equivalent Physician, by Months of Operation

	Number of Months of Operation			
Hospital	*1-12* *(n = 13)*	*13-24* *(n = 13)*	*25-36* *(n = 11)*	*37-48* *(n = 5)*
A	1,562	2,159	3,410	a
B	1,966	3,537	3,746	3,490
C	1,622	2,769	b	b
D	2,174	2,615	3,323	a
E	3,380	4,804	4,314	4,767
F	2,203	8,172	7,914	6,087
G	3,102	3,409	4,110	3,380
H	1,943	2,938	3,108	b
I	4,419	4,130	a	a
J	4,249	3,705	3,950	a
K	1,470	2,274	2,543	a
L	1,424	2,278	2,293	a
M	383	606	1,620	2,643
Mean	2,300	3,338	3,666	4,073
S.D.	1,173	1,790	1,630	1,360
Range	383-4,419	606-8,172	1,620-7,914	2,643-6,087

Note: Where necessary the data have been adjusted to reflect twelve-month operational periods.
[a]Data not available because hospital went off grant prior to completing operational period.
[b]Data not yet available for groups due to the length of time in operation.

The preliminary findings presented here do not allow firm conclusions to be drawn regarding the performance or effects of hospital-sponsored group practices. These must await further analysis of additional data on more sites. Even with additional data, it will not be possible to state definitively that hospital-sponsored group practice itself is responsible for or is the cause of whatever outcomes are observed. A number of other factors have been operating in the grantee sites over the course of the grant that make it difficult to isolate the effects of the hospital-sponsored group practice itself. However, a more complete data set and multivariate analysis will permit more rigorous examination of some of the preliminary findings reported here.

With the preceding caveat in mind, it appears that HSPCGPs can have a positive impact on improving the organization of access to care and, at the same time, further the hospital's involvement in providing general medical-care services to the community. Second, it appears that HSPCGPs can help a hospital maintain its institutional viability by contributing to the use of hospital inpatient and ancillary services. Finally, it appears that HSPCGPs can, after an initial start-up period, operate at a level of productivity and efficiency that makes possible the eventual achievement of financial viability.

Table 8-6
Group Operating Margin, by Months of Operation

Hospital	Number of Months of Operation			
	1-12 *(n = 13)*	*13-24* *(n = 13)*	*25-36* *(n = 11)*	*37-48* *(n = 5)*
A	-0.742	-0.654	-0.534	a
B	-0.736	-0.590	-0.507	-0.519
C	-0.652	-0.424	b	b
D	-0.610	-0.542	-0.274	a
E	-0.221	-0.016	-0.102	-0.043
F	-0.576	-0.195	-0.295	-0.294
G	-0.689	-0.533	-0.428	-0.308
H	-0.703	-0.563	-0.319	b
I	-0.225	-0.325	a	a
J	-0.573	-0.584	-0.320	a
K	-0.767	-0.583	-0.395	a
L	-0.673	-0.417	-0.207	a
M	-0.927	-0.895	-0.435	-0.074
Mean	-0.623	-0.486	-0.347	-0.230
S.D.	0.200	0.219	0.129	0.219
Range	-0.927--0.221	-0.895--0.016	-0.534--0.102	-0.519--0.043

Note: Operating margin provides a measure of revenue in relation to expenses. It is computed as follows:

$$\frac{\text{Net operating revenue} - \text{operating expense}}{\text{Operating expense}}$$

When deficit margin equals zero, net revenue equals operating expense; when revenues exceed expenses, deficit margin assumes a positive value.
[a]Data not available because hospital went off grant prior to completing operational period.
[b]Data not yet available for groups due to the length of time in operation.

Qualitative Factors Associated with Different Performance Outcomes

This final section of the chapter highlights some of the more important qualitative factors associated with the different performance measures. This information is drawn from the longitudinal case-study analysis described earlier. As information is still being collected and analyzed, what is presented should be viewed as preliminary. More complete information concerning the organization and development of groups in the CHP will be presented in future reports.[21]

In developing group practices, hospitals had to confront a number of major issues and problems that created uncertainty and made successful program implementation problematic. In many cases how these issues and problems were dealt with had a major effect on the development and performance of the groups. The most important qualitative factors associ-

ated with the different performance outcomes are summarized in table 8–7.
These include strong medical-director leadership, successful physician recruitment and retention, having the development of the group seen as
central to the hospital's overall mission, type of organizational design used,
and the degree to which the group experienced administrative and operational autonomy from the sponsoring hospital. It appears that these factors
interact in complex ways and have different effects on different performance
outcomes.

Strong medical-direct leadership appears to be one of the most important factors associated with successful group performance. Beyond the need
to organize the practice, provide essential administrative leadership, and
recruit physician staff, the group medical director is often called on to assist
the hospital in overcoming medical-staff opposition that might arise as a
result of the group's establishment. With rare exceptions, hospitals in
the CHP faced some degree of opposition from their medical staffs and
the medical community at large. Strong medical-director leadership played
a key role in helping to overcome medical-staff opposition where it occurred. The more effective medical directors tended to be older, respected,
established physicians who were selected from within the hospital's medical
staff.

A second issue facing the groups during their early developmental
period was the recruitment and retention of physicians. The primary characteristics differentiating the more successful from the less successful sites in
regard to physician recruitment and retention were the presence of a residency program from which the group could draw physicians and the personal and ongoing involvement of the medical director in recruiting. The

Table 8–7
**Summary of Qualitative Factors Most Associated with Different
Performance Outcomes**

Performance Outcomes	Factors Most Associated with
1. Strengthened hospital's ongoing involvement in primary care	Strong medical-director leadership "Professional" organization design Central to hospital's mission
2. Improved organization of access to primary care	Did not overestimate demand Successful physician recruitment and retention Strong medical-director leadership Central to hospital's mission
3. Positive impact on hospital financial viability	Successful physician recruitment and retention High autonomy Strong medical-director leadership
4. Financially viable group	Successful physician recruitment and retention Strong medical-director leadership Multispecialty, urban/suburban sites

majority of the successful case-study sites were sponsored by hospitals with associated residency programs that offered an excellent source of physicians for the group. In *none* of the less successful case-study sites was the medical director personally involved in recruitment in a significant way. In some of these sites the medical director did not exist until the second year of operation. In others, poor choice of medical director proved to be a hindrance to recruiting additional physicians.

A further important issue in the early planning and development of the groups was the degree to which they fit in with the goals and overall mission of the sponsoring hospital. Other investigators have noted the importance of seeing ambulatory-care initiatives as stemming from the organization's philosophy and being a central part of its identity.[28]

In general, those sites did well where the goals of the group fit in well with the overall mission of the hospital and its view of the future. However, the degree to which a group fit in with the hospital's overall mission was a necessary but not sufficient condition for a high-performing group. Among the case-study sites, nine of the thirteen groups fit in reasonably well with the hospital's mission and future plans. Where this occurred, essential support from the hospital facilitated the development and performance of the group. Nonetheless, three of these nine sites performed poorly on a number of dimensions. This indicates that a cultural fit between the goals of the group and the central mission of the hospital does not necessarily assure the group's long-run high performance.

The development of an organizational structure was yet another major issue faced by the groups during their initial developmental period. Hospital-sponsored primary-care groups have been characterized by three types of organizational structures: (1) a *simple structure* characterized by few services and few providers and a managerial subsystem that is only beginning to emerge; (2) a *machine structure* characterized by a close relationship between the clinical and administrative systems, a relatively high degree of vertical and horizontal differentiation and a high degree of formal plans and procedures; and (3) a *professional structure* characterized by highly developed professional services that are very loosely tied to the management subsystem and characterized by limited vertical integration and a high degree of professional differentiation.[29] Most of the thirteen case-study sites contained elements of all three structures, although one design or another tended to dominate.

In general, five sites were predominantly of simple structure design; four tended toward a machine structure; three are best characterized as a professional structure; and it is not possible to classify one site due to its unique nature. In general, groups with a simple structure design exhibited relatively poor performance, suggesting that this type of structure, which depends on one or two key people, is extremely vulnerable, particularly when these key people lack the necessary expertise, experience, and leadership. On the other hand, the site that could be characterized as having professional designs were judged to be high performers. Two enjoyed unusually competent medical directors who were widely respected by hospital administration and medical staff alike and could therefore successfully negotiate on behalf of the group. Thus, based on the experience of the case studies, it appears that hospitals initiating primary-care programs should give attention to professional values and interests and rely on medical-director leadership to provide the necessary lateral linkage with hospital administration necessary to achieve required levels of integration.

Finally, the important question of how closely the group should be linked with the hospital's organization, existing programs, and services—that is, how much autonomy the group should have—had to be addressed. This issue was particularly salient to the CHP grantees because of the fundamental differences between inpatient and ambulatory primary-care programs. How the grantees dealt with this issue appears to have been a key factor in the implementation of the program over time.

Autonomy is a multidimensional concept composed of functional and structural dimensions on the one hand and administrative and clinical dimensions on the other. *Functional autonomy* refers to the group's ability to exercise relatively independent control over its budgeting, personnel, purchasing, and related decisions. *Structural autonomy* refers to the formal organizational and reporting relationships between the group and the hospital. The less formal and hierarchical these relationships, the greater the degree of structural autonomy. *Administrative autonomy* refers to the group's ability to manage its own internal affairs without interference from hospital administration. *Clinical autonomy* refers to the ability of the physicians to develop their own principles of practice, refer to other specialists as they see fit, and admit patients based on their best judgment.

Six of the case-study sites granted their groups a relatively high degree of functional autonomy—both administratively and clinically. Typically, this meant that although the group generally followed the hospital's personnel policies, exceptions could be made, and, most important, the group had control over the hiring and firing of personnel. In regard to purchasing, the hospital set a relatively high dollar limit beyond which it required approval, and allowed the group to use its own vendors where that proved beneficial from a cost, quality, or volume viewpoint. Groups with autonomy also enjoyed considerable discretion in the development of monitoring of their budgets and typically did their own billing.

In the clinical area, groups with high autonomy had almost total freedom in regard to patient-care practices, referrals to other physicians, and hospital admissions. They also exerted a major influence on physician recruitment. In general, there were fewer marked differences in clinical functional autonomy among the groups. Most were allowed to develop their own internal practice patterns as they saw fit and to refer and admit patients freely.

Several points can be made regarding those sites granted a relatively high degree of autonomy from the beginning. First, the majority of these sites experienced little or no medical-staff opposition. In contrast, the sites that experienced little autonomy tended to have considerable medical-staff opposition. Second, sites with a relatively high degree of autonomy experienced few problems in physician recruitment and retention. In contrast, most sites with very little autonomy had significant recruitment and retention problems. The direction of causality is not clear, however. Successful recruitment and retention may enable a hospital to grant considerable autonomy to a group of physicians. On the other hand, a hospital structuring the relationship so as to allow considerable autonomy may be better able to recruit and, in particular, retain physicians. Based on the experience with CHP groups, the latter seems the more plausible explanation.

Last, it is important to consider the relationship between group autonomy and performance. In general, those sites that had a high degree of autonomy were high performers on most dimensions—ongoing hospital involvement; improvements in the organization of access to care; group financial viability; and a favorable financial impact on the hospital itself. However, two of the sites that enjoyed autonomy performed less well, experiencing low productivity and volume and eventually terminating hospital sponsorship. Unlike the successful cases, in both of these there was lack of medical-director leadership and, in one case, a lack of administrative leadership as well. This finding suggests an additional important consideration in examining the degree of autonomy, namely, the need for a minimum level of expertise, experience, and leadership within the group itself.

Thus, based on presently available information, the key to successful implementation of HSPCGPs appears to lie in strong medical-director leadership and successful physician recruitment and retention. Where these features do not exist, it is extremely important that the group be seen as central to the hospital's overall mission for it to succeed. Other factors such as organization design and degree of autonomy are also important but appear to flow from the preceding considerations with, for example, strong medical-director leadership being more commonly associated with a professional model of organizational design.

Summary

This chapter has described the Robert Wood Johnson Foundation's Community Hospital Program, outlined the design being used to evaluate the program, and presented some preliminary findings concerning the development and performance of groups involved in the program. While it is clearly premature to draw any conclusions, it appears that hospital-sponsored groups may be able to improve the organization of access to care in the community while promoting the hospital's continuing involvement in primary care. HSPCGP may also have positive financial benefits for the hospital, and the practices themselves may be financially viable in the longer run.

Future reports will provide more complete findings regarding the performance and effects of hospital-sponsored groups in the Community Hospital Program as more data on more sites become available. The behavioral model of hospital-sponsored primary-care group practice will be tested through multivariate analysis to determine which factors are associated with the different performance outcomes being examined. It is also expected that the case-study analysis will provide a more complete qualitative picture of the organizational development and performance of groups as additional information on the case-study sites is collected and analyzed. The results of these analyses should shed light on the factors (hospital, group practice, and community) most strongly associated with HSPCGP performance. These findings should be of interest to public policymakers, physicians, and administrators alike.

Notes

1. M. Roemer, "From Poor Beginnings, the Growth of Primary Care, *Hospitals* 49 (1975): 39–43.

2. N. Piore, "Problems and Opportunities for Hospitals in Primary Care," in *Community Hospitals and the Challenge of Primary Care*, eds., J. Bryant, A. Ginsberg, S. Goldsmith, M. Olendzki, and N. Piore (New York: Columbia University Press, 1975).

3. J.M. Redmond, "Apply Effective Fiscal Techniques to Improve Ambulatory Care," *Hospitals* 50 (1976): 93–95.

4. G. Katz and F. Hollander, "From Clinic to Group Practice," *Hospitals* 49, no. 5 (1975): 67–71.

5. M. San Agustin, L. Goldfrank, and R. Matz, "Reorganization of Ambulatory Health Care in an Urban Municipal Hospital," *Archives of Internal Medicine* 136 (1976): 1252–1266.

6. P.M. Ellwood and C.K. Ellwein, "Physician Glut Will Force Hospitals to Look Outward," *Hospitals* 55, no. 2 (1981): 81–85.

7. P.J. Feldstein, "Economic Success for Hospitals Depends on Their Adaptability," *Hospitals* 55, no. 2 (1981): 77–80.

8. S.J. Williams, T.M. Wickizer, S.M. Shortell, "Hospital-Based Ambulatory Care: A National Survey," *Hospital and Health Services Administration* 26, no. 4 (1981): 66–80.

9. S.J. Williams, "Ambulatory and Community Health Services," in *Introduction to Health Services*, eds. S. Williams and P. Torrence (New York: Wiley, 1980).

10. S.M. Shortell, W.D. Dowling, et al., "Hospital-Sponsored Primary Care: Organizational and Financial Issues," *Medical Group Management* 25, no. 3 (1978): 16–21.

11. S.J. Williams, S.M. Shortell, and W.D. Dowling, "Hospital-Sponsored Primary Care Group Practice: A Developing Modality of Care," *Health and Medical Services Review* 1 (1978): 1–13.

12. S. Ginsberg, S. Goldsmith, N. Olendzki, et al., *Community Hospitals and the Challenge of Primary Care* (New York: Columbia University Press, 1975).

13. D.M. Ambrose, "Primary Care Group Practice: Impact on a Community Hospital," *Hospital and Health Services Administration* 25, no. 2 (1980): 87–100.

14. J.N. Simpson, The Ashland plan: An ambulatory care outreach alternative for a community hospital. Hospital Administration 1975; 20: 33–53.

15. E.J. Sussman, H.M. Rosen, and A.J. Siegel, "Can Primary Care Deliver?" *Journal of Ambulatory Care Management* 2, no. 3 (1979): 29–39.

16. J.A. Block, D.P. Bourque, R.B. Froh, et al., "Physicians and Hospitals: Providing Primary Care," *Medical Group Management* 25, no. 2 (1978): 35–38.

17. J.A. Block, L.C. Brideau, A.K. Burns, et al., "Hospital-Sponsored Primary Care: The Community Hospital Program," *Journal of Ambulatory Care Management* 3, no. 2 (1980): 1–13.

18. N. Denzin, "The Logic of Naturalistic Inquiry," in *Sociological Methods: A Sourcebook*, ed. N.K. Denzin (New York: McGraw-Hill, 1978).

19. S.M. Shortell, T.M. Wickizer, N. Urban, et al., "Evaluation of Hospital-Sponsored Primary Care Group Practice: A National Demonstration," *Annals of the New York Academy of Sciences* 387 (1982): 69–90.

20. Fourth annual progress report to the Robert Wood Johnson Foundation, Center for Health Services Research, Department of Health Services, University of Washington, Seattle, Wash., March 1982.

21. S.M. Shortell, T.M. Wickizer, J.R. Wheeler, *Hospital-Sponsored Primary Care: A National Demonstration* (Ann Arbor: Health Administration Press, forthcoming, 1984).

22. J.R. Wheeler, T.M. Wickizer, S.M. Shortell, et al., "The Effects of Primary Care Group Practices on Community Hospitals" (Paper delivered at the 110th Annual Meeting, American Public Health Association, Montreal, Canada, November 14, 1982).

23. C. Brecher and M. Forman, "Financial Viability of Community

Health Centers," *Journal of Health Politics, Policy and Law* 5, no. 4 (1981): 742–768.

24. B.C. Campbell and E.K. Hudson, "Transformation of a Hospital Clinic to a Private Office Practice," *Journal of Ambulatory Care Management*, July 1978, pp. 2–8.

25. G. Sparer and A. Anderson, "Cost of Services at Neighborhood Health Centers," *New England Journal of Medicine* 286 (1972): 1241–1245.

26. B. Schultz, "An Analysis of Hospital Ambulatory Care Costs," unpublished Ph.D. dissertation, New York University, New York, 1975.

27. G.L. Glandon and R.J. Shapiro, eds., *Profile of Medical Practice 1980* (Chicago: American Medical Association, 1981).

28. T.B. O'Donovan, "The Primary Care Initiative: An Interview with Edward J. Connors," *Journal of Ambulatory Care Management* 4 (1981): 29–42.

29. A.D. Kaluzny and T.R. Konrad, "Organizational Design and the Management of Primary Care Services," in *Management of Rural Primary Care—Concepts and Cases* ed. G.E. Bisbee (Chicago: Hospital Research and Educational Trust, 1982).

9

Financing a Hospital-Sponsored General Medical Practice: The Beth Israel Ambulatory-Care Program

Michele S. Winsten,
Harvey J. Makadon, and
Thomas L. Delbanco

Ten years ago Beth Israel Hospital, a 452-bed university teaching hospital in Boston, organized one of the first hospital-based group practices in the country. The Beth Israel Ambulatory Care Center (BIAC) was created with three explicit objectives: (1) to develop a one-class primary-care practice serving, at reasonable cost, those who chose to receive their health care at Beth Israel Hospital; (2) to graft onto this system a program of education that would attract young health professionals into careers in primary care; and (3) to encourage both clinical and health-services research.[1,2]

Since attempts have been made to curtail spiraling health-care expenditures, which may reduce the access of many citizens to health care, it may be useful to examine the BIAC experience. Since cost issues are foremost among factors affecting outpatient units today, this discussion shall focus on both the hospital and society's perspective of the fiscal implications of a program such as BIAC. This discussion is presented in two sections: first, a brief description of BIAC today, including the delivery system, automated administrative functions, teaching and research; and second, an analysis of BIAC's financial picture.

BIAC Today

BIAC includes a general internal-medicine unit, an obstetrical/gynecological unit, and a walk-in unit. This chapter will consider only the first unit.

Delivery System

Patients receive ongoing health care in the BIAC medical unit from a team of health professionals that includes faculty physicians, residents and fellows in general internal medicine, nurse practitioners, social workers and

111

psychiatrists. There are four teams in the unit. Patients have twenty-four-hours-a-day, seven-days-a-week access to a physician. When hospitalized or referred to subspecialty units, patients are managed as private patients of their personal BIAC physicians. Mental-health care is integrated fully into the delivery system, with the BIAC psychiatric and social-service staff functioning both as direct providers and consultants to other team members. There is an active home-care program closely affiliated with BIAC; patients who require recuperative-facility follow-up remain under the care of the BIAC physician.

Today the medical unit manages approximately 6,000 patients with 22,850 visits annually on a fee-for-service basis. Patients vary in age from sixteen to one hundred and are drawn from a varied ethnic, socioeconomic, and residence base, as table 9–1 indicates. Visit charges vary by length of visit. They are comparable to other OPDs and private offices in greater Boston, and somewhat higher than those in many neighborhood health centers. Patients who have no third-party coverage and cannot afford to pay fully for their care pay reduced fees or make multiple-payment arrangements.

The medical unit includes nine faculty general internists, seventy house staff and fellows in general medicine, four nurse practitioners, five social

Table 9–1
BIAC Medical-Unit Patient Population

Patient or Visit Characteristics	Percent
Patient Age Distribution	
Over 85	2.1
76–85	7.8
66–75	12.7
56–65	12.9
46–55	12.8
36–45	14.6
26–35	23.4
16–25	13.7
Visit Primary Payment Source	
Self-pay	16
Medicaid	25
Blue Cross	27
Medicare	32
Patient Education	
Elementary	18
High school	59
College	23

workers, two part-time psychiatrists, and support and administrative staff. All except for the faculty are full-time employees of the hospital. The faculty internists hold full-time academic appointments at Harvard Medical School and are members of the Division of General Medicine and Primary Care in the Beth Israel Department of Medicine. The chief of the division is analogous to the chief of cardiology or nephrology. The faculty-group-practice arrangement is described later in this chapter.

Education Programs

The program of education in BIAC is varied and active. Students of medicine, social work, nutrition, and nurses training to become practitioners, work as apprentices to the nuclear faculty team of physician, nurse practitioner, social worker, and nutritionist. They join the practice to the extent that their training permits, participating in several teaching conferences that are held each week. In addition, all house staff in the Department of Medicine practice in BIAC at least one session per week during their entire three-year-residency experience, providing continuity of care to their patients. The faculty teams back up those house officers who are unable to manage their patients when other responsibilities intervene.

The Division of General Medicine and Primary Care is also responsible for much of the education of residents in a special track. The general-medicine residency is for house officers who wish to have an intensive experience in primary care and general medicine. After the traditional internship (PG 1) year, those who enter the general-medicine residency spend six months of each of the two subsequent years (PG II and III) in ambulatory care. Of the house officers in the Department of Medicine training program, 30 percent are in the primary-care track, and in recent years there have been more applicants from the hospital pool of interns than can be accepted for the program. Fellows in Harvard's Kaiser Fellowship Program in General Medicine also practice and teach in the unit.

Research Activities

Clinical- and health-services-research efforts have grown steadily in the program. Each of the faculty devotes at least 25 percent of their effort to research. Fellows join in studies in preparation for academic careers in general internal medicine. The faculty have published more than forty articles describing investigations undertaken within the program. Examples of topics of active inquiry include: clinical epidemiological studies of common infections, management of alcoholism by the general internist, interventions to improve functional status of the disabled, and factors influencing the practice of breast self-examination.

Automated Administrative Functions

Many of the BIAC clinical and administrative functions are computerized. These include a registration system that captures demographic data, the appointment-scheduling system, storage of clinical laboratory data and prescription information, and a provider-activity-information system. Health professionals use terminals located in each of the team-practice areas to review their schedules and retrieve data on their patients, including past admissions, clinical laboratory and radiographic reports, and medication profiles. When BIAC patients are admitted to the hospital, the physician is notified automatically by computer. The provider-activity-information system periodically generates a series of reports for the practice administration and individual practitioners describing the clinical activity of all BIAC faculty internists, residents, and nurse practitioners.

Financial Analysis

The hospital evaluates BIAC's fiscal status primarily on the basis of a pro forma that includes direct revenue, direct and indirect costs. "Indirect" revenues generated by grants, hospitalizations, ancillary tests, and referrals to specialists are considered separately. In the following discussion, we will describe the methodology used to generate the pro forma, to calculate BIAC's other sources of revenue, and to evaluate the effects of the hospital's contracts with various third-party payors. The analysis is included because it is crucial to understanding the hospital's perception of BIAC's costs and contributions. Moreover, the methodology itself may be useful to managers in other outpatient centers, even though such contracts will vary greatly in different states.

Until October 1982, the methodology described next applied. Starting in October, the prospective-reimbursement program described in chapter 5 on Blue Cross applies to *all* third parties in Massachusetts. A new state law mandates this change, and Medicare granted the Commonwealth a waiver permitting a trial of prospective reimbursement. This chapter outlines the convention that applied prior to October 1982 because it is broadly applicable to programs in other states, the majority of which remain under reimbursement conventions based on retrospective costs or charges.

Revenues from Clinical Services

The BIAC experience for clinical revenues and expenses is shown in table 9–2. *Gross revenue* is total actual patient-visit charges. This amount is derived from an encounter form used to generate patient bills.

Table 9–2
BIAC Medical Unit, Pro Forma
(fiscal year 1982)

Revenue (excluding grants)		
Gross Revenue		$810,000
Adjustments to gross revenue		
Bad debt and free care	($ 94,000)	
Contractual adjustments		
Medicare	$104,200	
Medicaid	($ 52,700)	
Blue Cross	$100,100	
Total contractual adjustments	$151,60	
Net revenue		$867,600
Direct expenses		
Salaries and wages	$506,400	
Fringe benefits	$ 96,200	
Payment to group-practice plan	$218,000	
Supplies and expenses	$ 37,500	
Total direct expenses		$858,100
Net after direct expenses		$ 9,500

Net revenue is calculated by adjusting gross revenue for bad debt and free care and for the hospital's contractual agreements with Medicaid, Medicare, and private insurance, which is primarily Blue Cross. Therefore the two factors that determine BIAC's net revenue are the BIAC patient payor mix and the details of the hospital's contracts with its third-party payors. The hospital's Fiscal Department performs numerous complex manipulations to derive the total hospital's net revenue. The bulk of these manipulations concern the inpatient areas. All outpatient activity is combined. Staff of the Fiscal Department and Ambulatory Administration have developed a simplified methodology to determine the net revenue generated by any single outpatient area. The following factors are included in the calculations.

Bad Debt and Free Care. This figure equals adjusted (free-care) and uncollected (bad-debt) charges. These charges include total charges billed to self-pay patients and the deductible and coinsurance portions of charges billed to third-party payors. Sixteen percent of BIAC medical-unit patient visits are self-pay.

Medicare. Thirty-two percent of BIAC medical-unit-patient visits are covered by Medicare. Medicare, prior to the Massachusetts waiver in October 1982, paid primarily on the basis of retrospective costs. In the outpatient units, Medicare was calculated as reimbursing 80 percent of total costs and 20 percent of charges (representing the deductible and coinsurance). Since bad debt and free care have already been accounted for, we assume 100 percent collection of the 20 percent charges. Because Medicare was cost based, and costs are higher than charges in the unit, the Medicare contractual adjustment became an *addition* to gross revenue.

Medicaid. Twenty-five percent of BIAC medical-unit-patient visits are covered by Medicaid. In Massachusetts, Medicaid reimbursement for outpatient units has been calculated on the basis of a cost/charge formula (two-year-old costs/one-year-old charges). Medicaid therefore reimbursed less than 100 percent of charges. Since costs are greater than charges in BIAC, the Medicaid contractual adjustment resulted in a *reduction* from gross revenue.

Blue Cross. Twenty-seven percent of BIAC medical-unit-patient visits are covered by Blue Cross. Effective FY 1982, the hospital signed a Blue Cross Maximum Allowable Cost (MAC) contract. The contract is based on two primary principles: The first limits growth in hospital expenditures through prospective reimbursement. Base-year costs for 1981 are adjusted for inflation to determine allowable costs in FY 1982, FY 1983, and FY 1984. The second principle provides an incentive to reduce inpatient volume and to increase outpatient volume. Thus, while prospective reimbursement limits costs that will be reimbursed, outpatient areas can increase revenues by increasing volume, if they maintain the same (or slightly higher) costs. The hospital is reimbursed 60 percent of unit costs for all outpatient volume above the FY 1981 base and loses 60 percent of unit costs for all decreases in volume more than 2 percent below the 1981 base.

An even stronger incentive is applied to outpatient ancillary volume. Here the hospital is reimbursed 100 percent of unit costs for up to a 2-percent increase in outpatient ancillary volume and 60 percent of unit costs for all volume increases beyond 2 percent. The hospital loses nothing for decreases in outpatient ancillary volume up to 5 percent and loses 60 percent of unit costs thereafter.

The MAC contract is applied to determine the Blue Cross contractual allowance in the following manner: The direct and indirect BIAC costs are calculated for FY 1981. This cost figure is then inflated by a MAC inflation factor specified by Blue Cross. Inflated costs are adjusted if there is a change in patient-visit volume. The volume calculation includes all visits to the unit, not only those covered by Blue Cross policies. When there is an increase in overall volume, as occurred in BIAC in FY 1982, costs are increased by 60 percent of the unit cost per visit for all visits above the FY 1981 visit volume. The reverse is true when there is more than a 2 percent decrease in visit volume.

The BIAC Blue Cross contractual adjustment for FY 1982 was an *addition* to gross revenue. This addition accrued from three factors. First, Blue Cross is a cost-based reimburser, and BIAC's costs *exceed* charges; second, BIAC's costs in FY 1982 did *not* exceed the 1981 base costs adjusted for inflation; and third, BIAC *increased* its volume in FY 1982 above the FY 1981 base.

As depicted in table 9-2, the BIAC aggregate contractual adjustment for FY 1982 was *an addition* to gross revenue of almost $152,000. While BIAC's gross revenue was $41.54 per visit, net revenue was $44.49 per visit. The positive contractual adjustments arose from two factors. First, both Medicare and Blue Cross reimbursed largely on the basis of costs (although Blue Cross was prospective), and BIAC costs exceeded charges. Second, 59% of BIAC patient visits are from these payor classes. These two factors are clearly crucial in maintaining BIAC's fiscal strength.

Revenues from Grants

The BIAC internal-medicine faculty generate approximately $500,000 per year in grant revenue for research and teaching. About 10 percent accrues to the hospital as overhead.

Direct Expenses

The hospital considers direct expenses to include salaries and wages, fringe benefits, supplies and expenses, and payments to the Department of Medicine for services rendered by the faculty. Salaries and wages include the salaries of all BIAC staff except the clinical portion of the faculty physicians' salaries. These are paid directly by the Department of Medicine. The department, in turn, is reimbursed by the hospital for each patient visit based on a group-practice arrangement, described later in this chapter. All medical housestaff salaries are prorated on the basis of time actually spent in BIAC. Fringe benefits are calculated at 19 percent, which includes the dollar cost to the hospital of life and health insurance, pension plans, workman's compensation, social security, unemployment insurance, and the costs of areas devoted to staff services.

"Silent" Revenues and Indirect Expenses

In addition to BIAC's direct revenue from patient visits, BIAC generates revenue for the hospital from inpatient admissions, referrals to specialists, and ancillary tests performed by the hospital laboratories. This is referred to as *silent revenue*, since hospitals may fail to recognize explicitly a practice's role in generating this income.

The value of this income to our hospital has changed dramatically over the last ten years. At the time of BIAC's inception, the hospital's inpatient facilities, ancillary services, and consultants were underused. Medicaid reimbursement covered close to 100 percent of charges; both Blue Cross and Medicare reimbursement were retrospective and cost based. Thus BIAC's ability to fill beds, refer patients to specialists, and order ancillary tests resulted in significant revenue for the hospital, and there was a clear and strong incentive for BIAC to generate as much silent revenue as possible.

On the other hand, from a perspective beyond the hospital's particular needs, one may view BIAC's activity in hospitalizing patients, ordering ancillaries, and referring patients to specialists as *cost* producing. As health-care expenditures grow at a rapid pace, policy analysts and legislators increasingly have become aware that hospital-based outpatient centers charge more than most neighborhood health centers and some private doctors' offices. Some have begun to question the necessity for this source of care. Thus our practice finds itself needing to both maximize silent revenues to maintain support from the hospital while wanting to minimize these same revenues to maintain societal support. This conflict was exacerbated by retrospective cost-based reimbursement, which created little incentive for the hospital to control its costs and, in addition, dictated step-down cost allocations, which fell on the outpatient department. BIAC's indirect costs, over which it has little control, were therefore high, adding to BIAC's overall expense to society.

The implementation of prospective cost-based reimbursement in October 1981 for all third parties in Massachusetts has begun to move incentives into line with both hospital and societal needs. As described in the discussion of the Blue Cross MAC contract, under prospective reimbursement the Beth Israel Hospital is reimbursed for adjusted-base-year costs and for variable costs associated with increased outpatient volume. This creates an incentive for the hospital to both contain costs and maximize outpatient volume. BIAC may therefore meet both hospital and societal objectives by maximizing outpatient activity and minimizing inpatient activity. Moreover, the hospital now has a high inpatient census, further reducing incentives for BIAC to hospitalize patients in order to generate revenues.

Some primary care physicians use office-visit fees as a "loss leader," while generating a large proportion of their income from ancillary tests (particularly those performed in the physician's office) and hospitalized patients.[3] These revenues help offset a physician's indirect expenses, and the hospital, by analogy, views the silent revenues generated by the BIAC practice as an offset to the indirect costs that are so difficult to quantify in the complex hospital program and accounting system. Most certainly, the indirect expenses generated by stepdowns developed for reimbursement purposes do not reflect the true indirect expenses of the unit. For the purpose of the pro forma, the hospital and BIAC administration have agreed to use a variable-indirect-cost figure for medical records, billing, general administration, and other overhead costs by which indirect costs amount to approximately 30 percent of total expenses. In negotiating the BIAC budget each year, the hospital tends to view the silent revenues as a full offset for the indirect costs.

Paying the Professionals

Starting in 1981, the hospital contracted with the Department of Medicine for physician services. Prior to 1982 the hospital paid the faculty physicians directly for their clinical activity. In 1981 the Department of Medicine entered into formal negotiations with the hospital to develop the Group Practice Plan for the BIAC faculty internists. The department and hospital agreed on a methodology whereby the hospital pays the department a predetermined dollar amount per patient visit (the visit fee), and the department pays the faculty salaries. Negotiations between the hospital and the department to determine the visit fee necessitated a careful financial analysis of the entire practice. The formula developed for this purpose is described in table 9–2. The hospital administration established the principle that the unit should break even after *direct* costs based on the direct revenues included in the formula. The maximum per-visit fee paid to the department is therefore that amount that results in breakeven after direct costs.

The agreement is designed to follow several specific principles. It includes visits generated by *all* providers (nurse practitioners, residents, and faculty internists). This maintains an incentive for the entire unit to increase activity rather than for one group to increase activity at the expense of another. Second, to reward providers as directly as possible, an arrangement was developed that enables nurse practitioners to benefit from increased activity while the hospital continues to pay their salaries. Third, all types of visits (that is, new patients, brief revisits, and so on) are converted into standard units to provide a standard basis for reimbursement. The standard unit algorithm provides an incentive to maximize new-patient visits rather than repeat visits in order to promote growth in patient panels and prevent inappropriate repeat use of BIAC services.

Problems and Prospects

The benefits that hospital-sponsored OPDs may hold have been described elsewhere in the literature.[4] They have the potential to serve both rich and poor in one setting. They offer easy access to complex technology and specialized care. They may be excellent educational settings, attracting young health professionals into careers in general health care. They may serve as important laboratories for clinical and health-services research.

These attributes may generate similar costs. Hospital-sponsored practices may be very inefficient, particularly in the academic center where service, teaching, and research requirements can come into conflict. The space in which they are located is frequently expensive and limited, and the laboratory support services are often slow and costly. The ready availability of expensive technology may result in overuse and high cost. The burden of illness carried by patients seeking care in such settings may be considerable and difficult to manage. All these factors, along with the stepdowns dictated by accounting and third-party conventions, may lead to high charges, which in turn may drive away all patients except those who lack other options.

The roles that OPDs have filled for hospitals and for society have changed dramatically over the last ten years. Evaluating their contributions and costs is complex and difficult. Much as we have learned from the experiences of practices like BIAC, important questions remain unanswered.

There is the central issue of OPD case mix, compared to private physicians' offices and neighborhood health centers.[5,6] Do some patients require the sophistication of a teaching hospital? How many? One out of four patients receive health care in an OPD or ER. What would happen if OPDs closed? Would patients then go to emergency units or to neighborhood health centers? Would private practitioners accept patients they have not served in the past? Would such physicians educate residents in their offices? What is the future need for general internists, and what contribution is made by teaching and conducting clinical research in hospital-based settings?

Answers to many of these questions may become clearer in the next few years. We are hopeful that the BIAC program will shed some light in this area. We have learned a great deal, have enjoyed working in such a practice, and are encouraged that many others now are reporting a similar experience.

Notes

1. A.B. Berarducci, T.L. Delbanco, and M.T. Rabkin, "The Teaching Hospital and Primary Care: Closing Down the Clinics," *New England Journal of Medicine* 292 (1975): 615–620.

2. T.L. Delbanco and J.N. Parker, "Primary Care at a Teaching Hospital: History, Problems, and Prospects," *Mount Sinai Journal of Medicine* 45, no. 5 (1978): 628–645.

3. S. Schroeder and J. Showstack, "Financial Incentives to Perform Medical Procedures and Laboratory Tests," *Medical Care* 16 (1978): 289–298.

4. T.L. Delbanco, "The Teaching Hospital and Primary Care," *Journal of Medical Education* 50 (1975): 29–38.

5. S.W. Fletcher, R.H. Fletcher, E.M. Pappius, and R. Rudd, "A Teaching Hospital Medical Clinic: Secondary Rather Than Primary Care," *Journal of Medical Education* 54 (1979): 384–391.

6. J. Lion and S. Altman, "Case Mix Differences Between Hospital Out-Patient Departments and Private Practice," *Health Care Financing Review* 4, no. 1 (1982): 89–98.

**Part IV
Choices of Ambulatory-
Care Settings**

10

What Should the Government Pay for, and Where?

Donald A. Young

The predominant health-policy issue of the day is the cost of health-services delivery. Congress and the executive branch of the government have indicated their determination to keep governmental expenditures for health services within acceptable limits. The policies chosen to contain costs may have a significant impact on the delivery of ambulatory services. Similarly, the shift from inpatient hospital care to ambulatory care may have a significant, but not always predictable, impact on costs. Changes in the nature of medical practice, technological advances, and service delivery require corresponding changes in governmental coverage-and-reimbursement policies, which in turn affect access to services, quality of care, and total costs.

For a number of years health-care financing has focused on the means and incentives to shift the delivery of health services from the inpatient hospital setting, which is considered very costly, to ambulatory-care settings where costs are less. The total cost savings of such policies is unclear, however. Hospital costs have continued to increase at a rapid rate[1] while costs and use of ambulatory-care services have risen at an even greater pace.[2]

Concurrent with the effort to move services out of the hospital have been dramatic changes in the way ambulatory-care services are organized and delivered. For example, prior to 1965 when the Medicare and Medicaid programs were authorized, the medical profession required many surgical procedures, now done on a daily basis in many ambulatory surgical centers, to be performed only in hospital inpatient settings. Far-reaching technological and research advances have further promoted the movement of services out of the hospital. Examples of such advances include the ability to deliver total parenteral nutrition in the home, home blood-glucose monitoring, digital venous angiography replacing the riskier arterial arteriography, and pumps for the infusion of drugs to treat cancer. Technological advances have also been associated with the emergence of commercial groups furnishing services in place of or in addition to traditional physicians' services.

On the policy side, Congress has responded to some of these changes by recently expanding ambulatory-services benefits and authorizing Medicare

The views expressed in this chapter are those of the author. No official support or endorsement by the U.S. Department of Health and Human Services is intended or should be inferred.

payment to free-standing ambulatory surgical centers and comprehensive outpatient rehabilitation facilities. In addition to authorizing these new benefits, Congress moved from traditional cost-based reimbursement for facility services and authorized payment on a prospective fee basis. At the same time Congress was expanding the array of ambulatory benefits, however, it also was indicating its concern with cost by authorizing the Secretary of Health and Human Services to set limits on reimbursement for services furnished in hospital OPDs, community health centers, and clinics as well as physicians practicing in these facilities.

Significant legislative change has also been made in the Medicaid program. These changes give increased flexibility to states regarding the reimbursement of hospitals, coverage of and services for the medically needy, authority to waive certain freedom-of-choice provisions for Medicaid eligibles and other provisions that have significant impact on ambulatory-care services.

This chapter will focus on ambulatory-care policy issues raised by the need for the Medicare and Medicaid programs to keep pace with the emphasis on cost containment, the significant technological and medical-practice innovations occurring, and the resulting changing pattern of service delivery. It must be emphasized, however, that Medicare and Medicaid are based on 1965 legislation that set the basic structure, benefits, and reimbursement methods for both programs.[3] Any future policy shifts must either be fit into this structure or be associated with significant legislative change as was the case with ambulatory surgery. Medicare and Medicaid, like most health-insurance programs, have historically paid for inpatient hospital care. Even though coverage of ambulatory-care services has grown, the bias toward the inpatient side has continued.

In the following discussion, it is important to make a distinction between public-policy issues related to *coverage* of services and issues related to *reimbursement* for services. A service must be covered as a benefit of the Medicare or Medicaid programs before issues of reimbursement come into play. Reimbursement in the terms of these programs means the methods and amounts of payment for services that are covered. For example, a new device may be developed that monitors the rhythm of the heart in a new and innovative way. Since heart-rhythm monitors are covered services, the policy issue becomes one of reimbursement. Should the level of reimbursement for the device be the same as for devices previously covered, or is there reason for a different level of reimbursement? Policy issues related to reimbursement will be considered in the next section.

The structure of the Medicare and Medicaid programs results in coverage-reimbursement policies that vary depending on the location of the service (hospital, doctor's office, clinic) or the characteristics of the individual or group furnishing the service (institutional provider, doctor, commercial group). With the exception of certain procedures and technologies that are not generally accepted or proven to be safe and effective, the Medicare program covers most services provided to hospital inpatients if the patient's medical condition and level of care are judged to warrant them.

Ambulatory-care benefits, while broad, are not as comprehensive as inpatient hospital benefits. For example, only those drugs and medicines that cannot be self-administered are paid for in ambulatory settings. Other procedures such as cardiac rehabilitation with exercise-stress testing, until recently have been covered only in the hospital (inpatient or outpatient) setting. Also, while physicians have always been paid for performing surgical procedures regardless of the site of the service, only hospitals could be paid a facility fee (or cost) for their component of the surgical service until the Medicare statute was changed with the addition of the ambulatory-surgery benefit.

Site-of-Service and Coverage Policy

Policy change to foster the movement of services to less costly settings is slow and at times uncertain. As changes in the patterns of service delivery occur, public policy may lag behind, leaving in place a system with incentives to foster inappropriate inpatient hospitalization for the purpose of receiving third-party reimbursement for costly procedures.

Redesigning benefit packages to keep pace with new technologies and alternative sites of service delivery will continue to be a major public-policy issue. While the case can be made to make such changes promptly, an alternative view advises caution based on quality and use concerns. Hospitals, including their OPDs, must meet certain health-and-safety standards to participate in the Medicare program. It is also generally assumed that either formal or informal peer review for quality and appropriateness of care is present in most hospital settings but lacking in many ambulatory settings.

A change in the site at which a service is furnished raises a host of policy decisions. When a device is used to measure a patient's blood sugar in the hospital, laboratory standards and certification assure that the measurement is accurate and meaningful to the care of the patient. Devices are now available for home blood-glucose monitoring. In the home setting, however, will the device give accurate and reliable measurements in the hands of relatively untrained individuals? Further, since the patient, with the advice of the physician, determines the frequency of measurement, there is the possibility of inappropriate use in both the frequency of testing and the types of patients acquiring the device. To the extent the use of such technologies in the ambulatory setting substitutes for or replaces hospital care, such devices result in decreased costs. To the extent they add new services that are not subject to requirements for utilization review, they may increase costs.

As new procedures and technologies emerge, the medical and scientific data base may be sufficient to begin applying and paying for the technology under carefully controlled circumstances while additional data and experience are gathered. In many cases a new service may be available and covered as a benefit only in hospitals. As more experience is gained, the service moves out of the hospital. At this point, the question of coverage may again be examined because new questions of safety and effectiveness arise as in the home blood-glucose-monitoring example or because of the differing policy rules for coverage of services in ambulatory settings. Such was the case with total parenteral nutrition, which was initially furnished only in a hospital and covered as a hospital service. The movement of this technology to the home setting is of special interest because of the high cost and the potential to expand the indications for its use. As noted previously, the usual quality-and-utilization controls assumed to exist in hospitals are not present in the ambulatory setting. Restricting such procedures to the hospital would only further increase costs, however. Existing coverage, reimbursement, and administrative policies have difficulty keeping pace with the spread of such technology and the growth in expenditures as procedures become ambulatory services rather than hospital services.

Public Interest in Benefits

Increasing public attention is also being paid to the difference in insurance benefits for inpatient versus ambulatory services. Commercial and industrial groups developing new procedures and devices are also becoming interested in the design of benefit packages. Benefit decisions greatly influence the research, development, and marketing strategy of these groups. An example of the convergence of new technology, commercial development, and marketing and medical practice is illustrated by an article in a trade newsletter[4] discussing the increasing sophistication of heart-monitoring instruments for use in ambulatory settings. The article noted that equipment sales will increase significantly in the next few years and that cardiac-monitor manufacturers should be aware of the marketing possibilities in commercial heart-scanning services in individual doctors' offices, as well as cardiac-rehabilitation centers. They went on to note that in recent years physicians have found that ownership of scanning instrumentation can provide a profitable business with strong tax benefits. Increasingly, public policy will have to take into account the growing influence of commercial and proprietary groups and the changing views of the medical profession regarding the business aspects of medical practice.

Very little attention has previously been given to technological change in the design of benefit packages in government-sponsored programs for delivery of health-services. With only occasional exceptions, services provided in hospitals are covered without much question, while more limited benefits are available in ambulatory settings. The movement of services out of the hospital coupled with technological change and continuing increases in costs, even in an ambulatory setting, will draw more attention to coverage policy and the need to set more coherent and consistent policies in ambulatory settings. Simply moving services from the inpatient hospital setting to the ambulatory setting, however, is unlikely to solve the problems of cost control.

Reimbursement and Changing Policies

Reimbursement policy for ambulatory services is complicated by the coverage-and-reimbursement provisions spelled out in the Medicare and Medicaid statutes. These programs have separate payment rules for provider services (including hospital and skilled-nursing-facility services) and for physicians and other health services. Under Medicare, inpatient hospital services are covered under hospital insurance and are paid for from the Part A trust fund. Outpatient hospital services are covered under supplementary medical insurance and are paid for from the Part B trust fund.[5] Both inpatient *and* outpatient hospital services, however, are paid for on a reasonable-cost basis. Physicians' services and "medical and other health services" are generally paid for on a reasonable-charge basis, even if the physician furnishes the service to a hospital inpatient. There are situations, however, in which the physician compensation is paid on a cost-related basis. Commercial groups providing services to ambulatory patients are also generally reimbursed on a reasonable-charge basis.

As a result of the structure of the Medicare statute, hospital-based ambulatory services are usually reimbursed on a cost basis while similar services furnished by nonhospital-based individuals and organizations are usually reimbursed on a charge basis. The need to classify services as either hospital or physician and other medical and health services creates inconsistency and at times incentives to the delivery of services that are not intended.

Classification of a service as a hospital service reimbursable on a cost basis (Part A) or as a physician or other health service reimbursable on a charge basis (Part B) determines amount of reimbursement, cost sharing (deductible and copayment), by the beneficiary, and choice of the site of service. The complexities in reimbursement policy introduced by the statutory requirement to pay for services based on the site of service rather than the nature of the service are further complicated by the previously mentioned changes in the organization and delivery of services. The policy problems and complexities are illustrated by the movement of surgical services to ambulatory settings.

The removal of a cataract provides an example of the variety of settings and reimbursement mechanisms currently available for a single procedure. In all settings, the physician performing the surgery receives a reasonable-charge payment. In all ambulatory settings, the physician also has the option of accepting assignment as payment in full, in which case the beneficiary has no copayment responsibility. If the surgery is performed on an inpatient hospital basis, however, the beneficiary is responsible for the 20-percent copayment and the physician is reimbursed only 80 percent of the reasonable charge. If the procedure is performed in a hospital as either an inpatient or outpatient service, Medicare will pay the facility the reasonable costs of furnishing the service minus any applicable cost sharing. If the procedure is done in a free-standing ambulatory-surgical center meeting Medicare's conditions of participation, Medicare will pay a prospectively determined facility fee without any beneficiary cost sharing. If the procedure is done in a physician's office, there is currently no overhead payment allowed beyond the physician's reasonable charge minus cost sharing by the beneficiary if the physician does not accept assignment. The bewildering array of payment mechanisms and amounts for the same procedure results from the complexity of the basic Medicare statute coupled with well-intentioned attempts to provide incentives to move surgical services from inpatient to ambulatory settings.

The Changing Role of Hospitals

The diversity of reimbursement alternatives, the expansion of hospital outpatient services, and increasing pressure on hospitals to constrain the growth of inpatient hospital costs has resulted in significant changes in the behavior of hospitals, which in turn will require adjustments in reimbursement policy.

As indicated in other sections of this book, many hospitals have diversified and become aggressive marketers of ambulatory services. Administrators have developed comprehensive outpatient services that effectively compete for patients with doctors' offices. While expanding outpatient services, hospitals have become sophisticated in applying the Medicare principles of reimbursement to maximize their cost-based reimbursement. As long as Medicare's reimbursement controls focus on inpatient hospital care, hospitals have an incentive to shift costs to outpatient departments. As Medicare-reimbursement policy catches up with this practice, hospitals may seek alternative means to maximize income. Since many ambulatory services may be covered and reimbursed as either hospital services on a cost basis or as other medical and health services on a charge basis, hospitals are exploring the possibility of altering their corporate structure to best fit their reimbursement needs.

Current reimbursement for hospital-based services is complex with patchwork changes being made on a regular basis. Such policy changes have a significant impact on both inpatient and ambulatory services. Deficiencies in cost-based reimbursement have been well chronicled. As a result, in recent years Congress has tentatively explored the area of prospective payment for facility services. The most notable examples of this trend are the legislative initiatives related to reimbursement for end-stage renal disease (ESRD) facilities and ambulatory-surgery facilities. Whether this trend will lead to major reform of reimbursement is unclear, but the notion seems to be gaining support.

Congress took a major step in this direction in the Tax Equity and Fiscal Responsibility Act of 1982 (TEFRA), P.L. 97–248. TEFRA directs the Secretary of the Department of Health and Human Services to develop a legislative proposal to put in place a system of prospective hospital reimbursement. At the same time Congress extended the so-called Section 223 hospital-cost limits to include the total operating costs of inpatient hospital services, including routine operating costs, ancillary costs, and special-care-unit operating costs. The new limits are to be applied on an average cost-per-case basis rather than on the prior per-day basis. In addition, the limits are to be adjusted for each hospital, based on the Medicare case-mix experience for that hospital. Since hospitals will be paid on a per-case basis, there is a strong incentive for hospitals to discharge patients earlier to outpatient settings and incentive, for those patients admitted to either provide some testing and other services on an outpatient basis prior to admission or after discharge. TEFRA also altered reimbursement for physicians practicing in hospitals and added new payment rules for some physician services furnished to hospital outpatients. The impact of these and other changes is only speculative now, but they provide strong incentives to shift the site of service from hospitals to other ambulatory settings.

The major policy issue relates to the use of reimbursement incentives, targeted to influence the behavior of hospitals and physicians. In the legislation establishing authority to pay for ambulatory-surgical services, a clear reimbursement incentive was given to Medicare beneficiaries to select free-standing ambulatory-surgical centers as their site of service with the requirement that the centers accept assignment for Medicare patients (thereby prohibiting the facility from billing the Medicare beneficiary for any additional charges). As a further incentive, the Medicare beneficiary is not required to pay the Part B deductible when the services are provided by an ambulatory-surgical facility.

Whether reducing beneficiary cost sharing will move services to ambulatory settings and reduce expenditures remains to be seen. To the extent that ambulatory services are less costly, savings may be realized. To the extent that absence of cost-sharing and utilization-review activities promote services that would otherwise not be used, the savings diminish. In addition, decreasing cost sharing also decreases revenues.

Physician Reimbursement

Physicians' services to Medicare patients are generally reimbursed on the basis of reasonable charges. The Social Security Act requires that payments must generally be made at 80 percent of reasonable charges to physicians for covered services. In determining reasonable charges, consideration is given to the customary charges generally made by the individual for similar services, as well as the prevailing charge in the area. In computing the reasonable charge, the Medicare program makes no distinction based on the location of the service (that is, physician's office or hospital OPD). However-er, the location of the service has an important bearing on whether the physician provides merely a professional service (that is, his own personal input) or whether there are also additional overhead costs associated with producing the services that the physician is personally responsible for.

For example, when a service is provided in the OPD of a hospital, Medicare reimburses the hospital for the facility costs, including rent, utili-ties, support staff, and supplies. When the physician provides the same service in the office, he is responsible for these overhead costs. Thus it is duplicative for Medicare to reimburse physicians for services in OPDs as if the physicians were responsible for the overhead expenses since the OPD is also reimbursed for these costs as part of the Medicare reasonable-cost-reimbursement process.

It is becoming increasingly necessary to distinguish between reimburse-ment for the physician's personal services and reimbursement for other overhead services. In 1965, when the basic Medicare-payment rules were established, payment for the services of a physician generally included limited resource inputs including an office, support personnel, and some supplies. For those occasional services that require more extensive inputs, for example, producing a complete electrocardiogram (EKG) as contrasted to simply interpreting the EKG, two different fees are recognized, one for only the professional component of the service and a larger fee for the total resource input.

Today, with technological changes and the movement of services from the hospital setting, services may include much larger resource inputs than the physician component. To complicate matters, the resource inputs may be provided by the hospital (which is reimbursed on a cost basis) or by other groups furnishing covered services and billing on a charge basis themselves. The policy problems include how to determine reasonable-payment levels, how to prevent duplicate payment when services are provided on both a cost and a charge basis, and how to prevent fragmentation and duplicate billing of charges by two or more individuals or groups. Significant reimbursement-policy issues also arise when new procedures are added to the list of covered benefits. While there are existing rules and procedures for determining the reasonable charge to be paid for such services, the rules may not meet the needs of all the parties-at-interest including those responsible for administering the Medicare and Medicaid programs.

The problem of determining an appropriate level of reimbursement revolves around the lack of a consistent definition of a unit of service for payment purposes and lack of data on which to judge the value and reasonableness of a service or the comparative value of components of services furnished by more than one physician specialist or other billing entity.

An example of this type of policy issue is shown with digital-subtraction angiography. This computer-assisted diagnostic-imaging test has been developed, diffused, and accepted by the medical profession over a relatively short time. The equipment is complex and expensive, but the procedure is relatively simple and safe. As a result, the procedure can be done in ambulatory settings whereas the procedure it replaced required hospitalization. The newness of the procedure and the high resource costs (especially the equipment) to produce the service present significant problems in determining a reasonable payment for the service on a charge basis. If the procedure were performed in the hospital, payment would include both reasonable cost to the hospital for the resource inputs and a reasonable charge to the physician for his contribution. In settings other than hospitals, however, a reasonable charge has to be determined for the total service.

While the medical profession has always held that physicians should determine their own usual charges, is it reasonable from a public-policy viewpoint to extend this tradition to procedures in which the physician's personal contribution may be a relatively small component of the charge? In cases such as digital angiography, the appropriateness of the charge may better be measured by the efficient and appropriate use of the equipment than by the contribution of the physician.

If traditional mechanisms for determining a fee are used and payment is too low in those situations in which the equipment is not efficiently used, physicians may have an incentive to increase use and bill for procedures that are not necessary. If the payment is too high, some physicians may receive rewards disproportionate to their contribution to the service. Similar problems have arisen in regard to payment of reasonable charges to suppliers of durable medical equipment, suppliers of nutrients for use in parenteral nutrition, commercial independent-laboratory services, transtelephonic monitoring of cardiac pacemakers, and many other services not furnished directly by physicians.

Problems and difficulties with both cost and charge-based reimbursement policy can be expected to increase as more technologically sophisticated services move from the hospital to other ambulatory settings and the financial gain in furnishing these services is increasingly realized by hospitals, physicians, and commercial groups.

Conclusion

The statutory requirements, changing pattern of ambulatory-service delivery, and the increasingly diverse settings in which these services are provided present immense administrative problems. The emphasis on restraining administrative, as well as program, costs requires tradeoffs that at times lead to policies that are flawed. It is important that those involved in health-services research, as well as those interested in coverage-and-reimbursement policy, develop a better understanding of the administrative needs and requirements of the programs as well as the influence of reimbursement policies on the patterns of service delivery.

Confronted with a statute, written in 1965 and changed at regular intervals, outlining basic rules for cost-and-charge reimbursement, those administering the Medicare and Medicaid programs, as well as Congress, have taken actions resulting in a patchwork quilt to cover and pay for the new array of services in emerging ambulatory settings.

The changes in site of service as well as the changes in the nature of hospitals and medical practice and the growing service role of commercial providers may be more than current statutory, regulatory, and administrative authorities and mechanisms can handle. It may no longer be possible to set coherent coverage-and-reimbursement policy on a case-by-case basis as was done with ambulatory surgery or use of medical equipment in the home.

Congress can continue to make minor incremental changes in benefits and reimbursement to keep pace with the changes in delivery of ambulatory services, or it can undertake a more fundamental reform of benefit structure and reimbursement for inpatient hospital as well as ambulatory-care services. Proposals for fundamental reimbursement reform are already on the public agenda. Whether restructuring of benefit packages will occur in conjunction with the reimbursement changes is less clear. The pressures to keep government expenditures, both program and administrative, in line while providing for the basic needs of Medicare and Medicaid beneficiaries require policy change of one form or another. The nature and impact of these changes on ambulatory services and the total cost of care remains to be seen.

Notes

1. Robert M. Gibson and Daniel R. Waldo, "National Health Expenditures, 1980," *Health Care Financing Review*, September, 1981.

2. George Schieber, "The Medicare and Medicaid Perspective," chapter 4 in this volume.

3. *Source Book of Health Insurance Data, 1980–1981* Washington, D.C.: Health Insurance Institute.

4. *Devices and Diagnostic Letter* 9, no. 123 (June 4, 1982): 2.

5. Schieber, "The Medicare and Medicaid Perspective."

11

Improving the Provision of Ambulatory Care by City Government: Preliminary Findings from the Municipal Health Program

Charles Brecher,
Ronald Andersen,
Edith M. Davis,
Gretchen V. Fleming, and
Miriam Ostow

Cities are major providers of ambulatory care, largely through health departments and public-hospital emergency rooms and clinics. The Commission on Public-General Hospitals reported that the ninety public-general hospitals found in the nation's hundred largest cities account for almost 30 percent of all hospital outpatient services in these cities.[1] Since low-income residents tend to rely disproportionately on public facilities, it is fair to conclude that city and county hospitals are a major source of ambulatory care for the urban poor.

However, there is widespread dissatisfaction with the way in which public hospitals in urban areas deliver services.[2] Among the most frequent criticisms are the relatively high cost and the fragmented character of outpatient care as well as the neglect of preventive services. In order to provide a model for improved delivery of ambulatory care by municipalities, the Robert Wood Johnson Foundation together with the U.S. Conference of Mayors and the American Medical Association launched the Municipal Health Services Program (MHSP). The purpose of this chapter is to describe the MHSP and the accompanying evaluation of the program and to present selected preliminary findings from the evaluation.

The Nature of the Municipal Health Services Program

In 1978 the Robert Wood Johnson Foundation initiated the MHSP as a national demonstration to assist cities in improving and expanding the health services they provide in underserved neighborhoods. The mayors of the fifty largest U.S. cities were invited to submit proposals for funding under the program. Of twenty-eight cities completing applications, five were awarded grants: Baltimore, Cincinnati, Milwaukee, Saint Louis, and

San Jose. The awards, made in June 1978, provided $3 million to each of the cities over a five-year period. The program is administered for the Robert Wood Johnson Foundation by The Johns Hopkins Hospital.

Program Objectives

Like many health-care demonstrations, the MHSP has three objectives: to *improve access* to care for the urban poor, to *improve the quality* of ambulatory care provided under public auspices, and to *reduce the costs* of care for clients of municipal health facilities. The MHSP seeks to promote these objectives by altering the structural arrangements for the delivery of care that prevail in most large cities.

The specific structural alteration is the creation or expansion of neighborhood-based ambulatory-care centers to serve populations that have historically been treated by public-hospital OPDs. These centers are to have referral arrangements for specialty and inpatient care at the city's public hospital. Preventive services of the local health department and traditional outpatient medical services of the municipal hospital are to be brought together in single neighborhood locations. The elected local officials, in cooperation with the heads of the municipal hospital and public-health department, are to be responsible for the design and implementation of the structural changes.

This strategy of shifting the locus of ambulatory care to neighborhood health centers under municipal auspices is axiomatic to each of the program objectives. Access should be improved by bringing primary-care services physically closer to clients at decentralized sites. In addition, community advisory boards are to be established for the centers in order to increase consumers' awareness of service availability. With respect to quality, municipal-hospital outpatient clinics are generally seen as impersonal, fragmented, overspecialized, and discontinuous sources of care. Similarly, traditional public-health departments are criticized for providing fragmented care divided along categorical program boundaries. The MHSP seeks to improve quality by offering comprehensive primary care for all family members at one location with referral linkages between the clinics and the municipal hospital.

Several features of the neighborhood clinics' operations are intended to advance the goal of reduced cost. First, costs should be reduced by freeing primary care from the expensive hospital overhead. Further savings should accrue from greater use of preventive services and from the substitution of ambulatory for inpatient care in appropriate situations. Finally, an emphasis on managerial efficiency at the neighborhood clinics should result in economies.

For readers informed about the history of the federally funded neighborhood health centers, this strategy and set of objectives should sound familiar. Through a series of programs beginning with the Office of Economic Opportunity's Community Action effort and continuing through the current Department of Health and Human Services' Community Health Center program, the federal government has funded several hundred neighborhood clinics.[3] However, the MHSP differs from these earlier efforts by virtue of its close ties to city government and mayoral leadership. The federal programs have relied primarily on private, nonprofit community groups as clinic sponsors, with these organizations frequently in political conflict with local elected leaders. The MHSP avoids such difficulties by working directly with City Hall, although community groups can be and are involved in the program. Moreover, the MHSP places considerable emphasis on efficient management while federal centers have been criticized for high unit costs and failure to collect maximum third- and first-party revenues.[4]

Waiver Component of the MHSP

In addition to benefiting from the Robert Wood Johnson Foundation's financial support, the MHSP clinics also are eligible for waivers of certain Medicare and Medicaid regulations under a parallel Health Care Financing Administration (HCFA) demonstration program. The purpose of the Medicare- and Medicaid-waiver demonstration is to see whether long-run savings will accrue to the federal government from shorter-run investment in "free" preventive and ambulatory services at neighborhood clinics. Improved access to such services is hypothesized to reduce the use of more costly specialist services and of hospitalization, thereby reducing the total annual cost per patient.

The Medicare waiver, which applies in all MHSP clinics, eliminates the coinsurance and deductible requirements under Part B; offers coverage for preventive and diagnostic services as well as drugs, eyeglasses, and dental care; and provides for clinic reimbursement on a cost, rather than comparable physician fee, basis. Each city's Medicaid waiver is different, generally covering preventive services not otherwise included and permitting cost-based reimbursement for clinics. The latter provision is particularly important in Missouri and Maryland, where regular state Medicaid programs pay clinics on a relatively low fee-for-service basis. In contrast, Cincinnati did not require a waiver because Medicaid reimbursement in Ohio was already cost based.

Design of the Program Evaluation

In keeping with the dual (Robert Wood Johnson Foundation and HCFA) nature of the MHSP, two complementary evaluations are being conducted.

The Center for Health Administration Studies (CHAS) of the University of Chicago is studying changes in use and cost resulting from enrollment in the MHSP clinics and from availability of the Medicare and Medicaid waivers. The Conservation of Human Resources (CHR) of Columbia University is documenting the process of change in the organization and financing of municipal health services accompanying implementation of the MHSP with the objective of determining the desirability and feasibility of similar changes by a greater number of cities. It should also be noted that the cities themselves in the course of their management functions perform a variety of evaluative activities and that the Foundation's program administrators at Johns Hopkins also monitor the progress of the demonstration sites. In fact, the administrative reports required of MHSP clinics were designed in a collaborative effort of the CHAS, CHR, and central administrative staffs.

In essence, the CHR evaluation seeks to ascertain whether the necessary structural change for program implementation occurs, what the obstacles are to such change, and what organizational, fiscal, and political factors contribute to long-run viability for MHSP clinics. The focus is on implementation within the distinct economic and political milieu of each city. The methodology adopted for this analysis is a monitoring approach developed by Richard Nathan for his evaluation of the revenue-sharing program for the Brookings Institution.[5] This approach combines a core staff based at CHR with a group of university-based field associates in each city. The CHR staff has devised uniform reporting protocols and relies on the field associates for the tasks of continuing observation, data gathering, and preliminary analysis. The field associates are drawn from sociology, public-health, political-science, and health-administration fields.

The evaluation of the MHSP undertaken by CHAS seeks to determine the effects of the Medicare and Medicaid waivers and MHSP clinic organization on access to services for the target population and on the total expenditures for care on behalf of this population. Since a major goal of the Health Care Financing Administration in testing the waivers is to realize economies in the total cost of providing services to the urban poor, the CHAS evaluation will compare total costs on behalf of MHSP clinic users with those of similar urban residents who do not use the MHSP clinics.

The methodology for the CHAS evaluation is a two-stage telephone survey in the service area of one MHSP clinic in each study city conducted at the outset of the program and three years into the program (August–November 1982). The telephone surveys provide information on the respondents' health status, health-service-use patterns, health-care expenditures, and socioeconomic status. Of particular concern are usual source of medical care for respondents, patterns of use of care, and costs (out-of-pocket and third-party) of health services consumed. In addition to the data generated through the two phases of the survey, information is also being gathered from Medicare- and Medicaid-claims files and MHSP clinic and public-hospital records.

Preliminary Findings

While neither element of the MHSP evaluation is completed, both are being conducted in stages that permit a presentation of preliminary findings. The CHAS team issued a report on its baseline survey in March 1982. An interim report will be issued during 1983, and a final report is expected in 1984. The CHR team has prepared a baseline volume titled *Health Care for the Urban Poor: Directions for Policy*, 1982, available from Allanheld, Osmun and Company. A final report will be prepared for publication late in 1983.

CHAS Preliminary Findings

The following are what we consider to be some of the most interesting findings in the CHAS baseline report.

1. *The target population of public-hospital and health-department clients is a relatively small proportion of the residents in the demonstration areas* (see table 11–1). Within the MHSP clinic-catchment areas in the five cities, the share of the surveyed population relying on the public hospitals for ambulatory services ranged from 2.2 percent to 18.7 percent. Surprisingly, a far larger share of the population in the MHSP clinic areas relies on private physicians for care. Among the five cities, this proportion ranged from 46.1

Table 11–1
MHSP Clinic Neighborhood Residents by Regular Source of Care
(*percent distribution*)

| Regular Source of Care | City (Percent) | | | | |
	Baltimore	Cincinnati	Milwaukee	Saint Louis	San Jose
Municipal hospital[a]	9.3	10.6	2.2	18.7	7.2
Private physician	56.8	70.6	59.7	46.1	64.0
Other hospital	14.3	5.4	14.0	15.6	6.0
Other source	4.6	2.7	8.4	3.9	6.9
No regular source	15.0	10.7	15.5	15.7	16.0
Total	100	100	100	100	100

Source: "Evaluation of Municipal Health Services Program, Phase I (Baseline) Study Report," HCFA-500-78-0097, Center for Health Administration Studies, University of Chicago, 1982.

[a]Includes MHSP clinic.

percent to 70.6 percent. Moreover, in every city, users of private physicians represent the largest single category.

2. *Public-hospital users differ from the balance of the population in the surveyed neighborhoods in the directions one might expect.* More public-facility users were minority and low-income citizens; their reported health status was poorer; and they tended to use health services less often than reported symptoms indicate they should.

3. *Public-facility users receive medical services (ambulatory and inpatient) at about the same rate as groups with other regular sources of care.* While there was substantial variation in use rates among the five cities, within each city there was a general similarity in use between public-hospital users and other area residents. Specifically, the range in physician visits among the cities was between 4.79 and 6.65 annually for all area residents, and between 4.27 and 6.91 for public-facility users. With respect to inpatient use, the number of hospital nights ranged from 0.69 to 1.73 annually for all area residents, and from 0.65 to 1.94 for public-facility users (see table 11–2).

4. *Total annual expenditures for medical care among public-facility users were generally lower than total medical-care expenditures among those whose regular source of care was a voluntary hospital and were quite similar to total medical-care expenditures among those who relied on private physicians for care* (see table 11–3). Again there was considerable variation among the cities: total per-capita expenditures varied from $691.80 to

Table 11–2
Use of Health Services among MHSP Clinic Neighborhood Residents, by User Status

	Reported Health Services Use	
City	Physician Visits	Nights in Hospital
Public facility users		
Baltimore	5.77	1.41
Cincinnati	5.97	0.90
Milwaukee	6.20	1.54
Saint Louis	6.91	1.94
San Jose	4.27	0.65
All respondents		
Baltimore	5.90	1.46
Cincinnati	6.65	1.38
Milwaukee	5.67	1.42
Saint Louis	6.25	1.73
San Jose	4.79	0.69

Source: "Evaluation of Municipal Health Services Program, Phase I (Baseline) Study Report, "HCFA-500-78-0097, Center for Health Administration Studies, University of Chicago, 1982.

$854.12 annually. But the relationships among costs for groups with each type of regular source of care were relatively consistent. Total costs were higher for voluntary-hospital users than for public-hospital users in four of the five cities by between 9 and 68 percent. In contrast, residents reporting public hospitals and private physicians as their regular source of care had annual expenditures that were quite similar in each city.

5. *The users of public facilities report a lower degree of satisfaction with the care they receive than do users of private physicians or users of voluntary hospitals.* Generally, residents relying on private physicians reported the greatest satisfaction, and voluntary-hospital users reported levels of satisfaction between those of public-facility and private-physician users. Of the aspects of care with which public-facility users were dissatisfied, the most troublesome were considered to be the nonmedical dimensions of access such as travel and waiting time. These criticisms are related to organizational factors that appear to be amenable to improvement via the structural changes incorporated in MHSP design.

CHR Preliminary Findings

The monitoring activities of the CHR staff, supplemented by operating and financial reports from the MHSP program administration, provide substantial information on the progress of the demonstration. The major findings to date are:

1. *Local governments participating in the demonstration program evidence a considerable commitment to structural change in the public health-care-delivery system.* The basic premise of the MHSP, that seed money could stimulate local-government initiative to shift services for ambulatory pa-

Table 11–3
Per-Capita Expenditures for Health Services among MHSP Clinic Neighborhood Residents, by Source of Care

Regular Source	City				
of Care	Baltimore	Cincinnati	Milwaukee	Saint Louis	San Jose
Public					
facility	783.11	604.03	942.58	926.12	648.48
Other					
hospitals	954.41	1004.62	795.38	1011.14	1087.55
Private physician	700.25	723.47	885.00	835.55	687.82
No regular					
source	49.55	51.57	87.88	186.04	85.94
All	731.61	705.44	854.12	847.65	691.80

Source: "Evaluation of Municipal Health Services Program, Phase I (Baseline) Study Report," HCFA-500-78-0097, Center for Health Administration Studies, University of Chicago, 1982.

tients from the public hospital to neighborhood clinics, has essentially been confirmed. Each participating city has opened the required number of clinics, and these facilities provide a significant number of visits. In the fourth year of the demonstration, the MHSP clinics provided over 218,000 visits. Based on comparisons with predemonstration public-health-department clinic activities, the MHSP administrators have estimated the increment in services generated by the program to be approximately 130,000 visits.[6]

2. *Due to a variety of factors, it has taken longer than expected to establish the MHSP clinics.* First, in many cities conflict arose among local agencies and citizen interest groups over site selection, and their resolution necessitated lengthy negotiations. It also required time and astuteness for program sponsors to assemble necessary capital funds for the facilities. The MHSP seed money did not include construction funds, so sources such as Community Development Block Grants were "packaged" by the cities for the program. Third, difficulties arose in staffing the clinics. In several cities the complexities of civil-service regulations and limited salaries meant delays and obstacles in recruiting and hiring the appropriate administrative and professional staff. These obstacles and other constraints led to considerable staff turnover in the clinics but also fostered creative arrangements for physician staffing at some sites. It should be noted that the initial expectation that staff would be redeployed from the public hospital to the clinics generally was not realized; most program staffing represented an add-on to preexisting personnel.

3. *It has proved difficult to achieve viable levels of use at new facilities.* Some clinics found themselves overstaffed for the available workload but could not cut back physician hours without leaving major services uncovered. The target volume of 4,500 visits annually per full-time-equivalent physician has not been reached at most clinics. Program managers perceive that the clinics have entered a competitive arena, and most sites are developing marketing techniques to attract a larger clientele. The Medicare waiver, which was anticipated to be a major marketing device as a result of its expanded range of no-charge services to beneficiaries, has drawn elderly clients to many of the clinics. However, the impact of the waiver has varied considerably across sites with the Medicare-patient load ranging from 3 to over 50 percent of total charges among the MHSP clinics.

4. *The low levels of use (and other factors such as construction, equipment, and other start-up costs) have kept unit costs higher than anticipated.* However, in most cases the cost per visit is below the public-hospital cost, and in the majority of cities it is near the program administrators' target of two-thirds the cost of a comparable public-hospital outpatient visit.

5. *A central goal of the MHSP, improved continuity of care through a strong link between the clinics and the municipal hospital for back-up spe-*

cialty and inpatient care, has not been achieved thus far in any of the cities. In most cities major obstacles were posed by the lack of admitting privileges at the public hospital for clinic physicians and by a general lack of organized contact between the two sites. Consequently, an unexpected development in the program has been the establishment of back-up linkages between the MHSP clinics and some voluntary hospitals in the service area. This has occurred in three of the five cities. This trend represents a major departure from original program goals, but at the same time signals a high degree of adaptability among the clinics.

6. *The outlook for financial viability of the clinics is a major concern.* Entering their fourth year, the MHSP centers were far from self-supporting. Operating revenues as a share of expenses averaged 55 percent and ranged from 20 to 90 percent.[7] Since the Robert Wood Johnson Foundation (RWJF) subsidy ends after the fifth year, city treasuries will be challenged to sustain the centers. At the same time the external funding environment is hostile and becoming worse. Both federal and state commitments to funding for health services are eroding under the pressures of a weakened economy, potential budget deficits, and a shift in intergovernmental definitions of responsibility. The survival of MHSP clinics will depend on the importance attached by the local political leadership to keeping the sites in operation.

Conclusion

These preliminary findings present a mixed picture of the success of the MHSP in attaining its objectives. We expect the outcome to be somewhat clearer when the final results are known, particularly the findings from the second round of the CHAS social survey. However, even then we will not be able to report the full extent of MHSP impact due to the complexity of the program, its interaction with a changing environment, and the inability to assess its long-term consequences until some time has elapsed after termination of the RWJF grants and the HCFA waivers.

Notes

1. Commission on Public-General Hospitals, *The Future of Public General Hospitals* (Chicago: Hospital Research and Education Trust, 1978).

2. For a review of the literature, see Eli Ginzberg, Michael Millman, and Charles Brecher, "The Problematic Future of Public General Hospitals," *Health and Medical Care Services Review* 2, no. 2 (summer 1979).

3. See Karen Davis and Cathy Schoen, *Health and the War On Poverty:*

A Ten Year Appraisal (Washington, D.C.: Brookings Institution, 1978), chap. 6.

4. See Charles Brecher and Maury Forman, "Financial Viability of Community Health Centers," *Journal of Health Politics, Policy and Law* 5, no. 4 (winter 1981): 742–768.

5. Richard Nathan, Allen D. Manuel, Susannah E. Calkins, and Associates, *Monitoring Revenue Sharing* (Washington, D.C.: Brookings Institution, 1975), esp. pp. 317–325.

6. Carl J. Schramm and Gary A. Christopherson, *Municipal Health Services Program Annual Report 1980–1981* (Baltimore: Johns Hopkins University, 1981) table 2, p. 4.

7. Ibid., tables C.1 and C.2, pp. 26–27.

12 Health-Maintenance Organizations and Medicaid

Howard R. Veit

The Medicaid provisions of Public Law 97–35, the Omnibus Budget Reconciliation Act of 1981, have provided state governments with greater latitude to develop innovative contractual arrangements with health-care providers to deliver prepaid health services to Medicaid recipients.

The new legislation enables states to enter into various reimbursement arrangements with organized groups of providers with the objective of providing high-quality services at a reduced cost to states. In broadening the definition of prepaid providers, Congress has recognized that prepaid care can be provided at lower cost, but that conventional health-maintenance organization (HMO) service capacity is currently insufficient to meet the needs of the states for lower-cost-provider options. Congress has also taken a step away from previous federal policy that restricted federal involvement in prepaid health care to qualified HMOs. Whether this policy shift has merit remains to be seen. One has only to be reminded of the "Medicaid-Mill" HMO scandals in California to become concerned about public policy that steers Medicaid recipients en masse into prepayment arrangements.

The new legislation encourages Medicaid contracts with prepaid providers or with organizations that (a) make covered services to Medicaid enrollees accessible on the same basis as the other Medicaid beneficiaries and (b) make provisions against the risk of insolvency. The legislation also allows the Department of Health and Human Services (DHHS) to waive some traditional Medicaid requirements such as recipient freedom of choice in order to allow the states to implement a primary-care management system, require individuals who overuse services to use particular providers, limit the participation of providers who have abused the program, and purchase directly (by competitive bid) special services such as laboratory and x-ray services.[1]

It is too soon to judge whether provider groups such as case-management organizations, primary-care networks or community health centers will be able to lower costs and assure the state that recipients will have adequate care. This author admits at the outset to a strong bias toward the health-maintenance organization that has most, if not all, of the characteristics of a federally qualified HMO, as the most appropriate delivery vehicle to provide prepaid comprehensive Medicaid benefits to an enrolled population. An HMO must be tightly organized, businesslike, and possess highly motivated providers in order to accomplish substantial cost reduction in the provision of health services. Living within prepaid capitation income is not easy and will not succeed unless unusually strong provider commitment exists.

The purpose of this chapter is to share both the opportunities and practical problems that HMOs have had with state Medicaid contracts in the hopes that these experiences will be useful to HMO, HMO-like, and non-HMO providers who dare venture forth into capitation (risk) contracts with states to serve Medicaid recipients. HMOs have traditionally not served the poor or the elderly in great numbers, although they are fully capable of doing so.

In this chapter *health-maintenance organizations* are defined as those organized systems of care (Individual Provider Associations or group practices) that *provide* comprehensive hospital and ambulatory medical-care benefits for a fixed, prepaid premium to a voluntarily enrolled population. They may or may not be federally qualified. The term *prepaid health plan* is used as synonymous with HMO.

The Growth of HMOs

Since 1970 there has been an increase in both the number of HMOs and the number of enrollees being served by them. In 1970 there were about 30 plans serving 3 million people. Today, there are 243 programs serving over 10 million.[2] This growth is a result of the federal government's strong advocacy of the concept of prepaid health care together with increased marketplace acceptance of this form of health-care delivery.

While a greater percentage of members are still in a relatively small number of programs that have been in existence for many years, most plans are small and developing, and their enrollments are increasing. Total enrollment has increased at an average annual rate of about 10 percent since 1978, so HMOs may eventually become a major provider of health services. Although the federal HMO effort has dwindled as a result of budget cuts that began in 1980, there is promise that private investors will provide capital to offset the loss of federal dollars for prepaid-plan development and planning. Although nonprofit programs are now and will probably continue to make up the majority, current trends indicate that there will be more Blue Cross plans and commercial insurance companies involved, more for-profit companies established for the purpose of investing in prepaid-plan development, and more for-profit programs.

The growth of prepaid plans is a significant development for government purchasers of health services. Although to date these plans have served mainly an employer group-based population, some programs do serve Medicare and Medicaid recipients. While less than 4 percent of pre-paid-plan enrollment is made up of Medicaid recipients,[4] where such factors as accessibility and member satisfaction have been measured, the results have been favorable. Fuller and Patera[5] and Gaus[6] have found that Medicaid enrollees rated HMO service as good, or better than, fee-for-service sources of health care. Other studies by Columbo[7] and Colton[8] have shown that HMO enrollment does not guarantee appropriate use of ambulatory services but such sectors as health education and outreach services have a positive impact on use of needed health-care resources.

Research that has looked specifically at Medicaid enrollment in HMOs has generally concluded that they provide Medicaid benefits at a lower cost than do traditional fee-for-service providers.[9,10]

Factors that Make HMOs Successful

For prepaid plans to be a significant factor in the provision of services to public beneficiaries, their growth must proceed as previously predicted so that financially sound programs are made accessible to the poor and the elderly. Only financially sound programs should be given contracts to serve public beneficiaries.

Some poorly conceived and/or managed plans have failed during the past few years and in the mid 1970s. California had a much-publicized scandal regarding prepaid plans that served a predominantly Medicaid population. Broad experience with prepaid plans, however, suggests that they can be financially sound in most urban areas if there is sufficient start-up and operating-deficit capital, good management, the establishment of effective business relationships with providers, and sufficient market-place acceptance.

Broad market acceptance is critically important to success. Plans must attract people who would ordinarily have chosen traditional health insurance. For a plan to compete successfully in the health-benefits marketplace, it must offer coverage that is the same or less in premium cost (even though plan coverage is usually more comprehensive), it must be easily accessible to its enrollees through conveniently located facilities, and it must have a reputation for high-quality services.

Prepaid plans achieve competitively priced premiums by effectively managing the provision of health services to their members and by effectively managing and investing their available cash. There are many examples of plans that have premiums lower than their competitors (Blue Cross and Commercial Insurance) while offering benefit packages that are much broader with fewer copayments and deductibles.

A key element in the HMO's ability to control costs is the prepayment incentive coupled with efficient organization and good medical management. Reimbursing providers on a capitation rather than a fee-for-service basis will result in lower costs over the long run only if the providers are sufficiently motivated to alter traditional patterns and to work an environment in which their colleagues will have a substantial amount of influence over both the quality and the economic aspects of their practice. In addition, providers must be able to accept the prepaid capitation amounts.

Plans that market a price-competitive premium must reduce levels of hospital admissions for their membership substantially below comparable populations in the fee-for-service system. This is the way plans accomplish most of their savings.[11] They must also control patient length of stay and control hospital per-day costs as much as possible. Finally, HMOs must control the costs of ambulatory care by maintaining optional ratios of providers to members and efficiently purchasing ancillary services and other types of services.

HMOs are, of course, affected by the rising costs of health services in the rest of the system. Rising hospital costs are of great concern especially in areas where they compete with a Blue Cross Plan that enjoys substantial contractual discounts with hospitals. In Philadelphia, for example, the Blue Cross Plan receives discounts of at least 20 percent off hospital charges. It is difficult for prepaid plans to obtain such favorable rates.

Although it is quite clear that hospital costs are substantially lower in HMO settings, comparative ambulatory costs are less clear.[11] HMOs do not normally calculate ambulatory-care costs in the same manner as other providers. The basis for calculating revenue to a fee-for-service provider is to multiply the cost per service times the volume. Income per visit related to cost per visit is significant. The prepaid plan, on the other hand, both insures and delivers a broad range of services that include hospital and ambulatory care. Since income is based on a prepaid premium from an enrolled membership, cost per member becomes the significant variable. Wherein fee-for-service providers have an incentive to maximize visit volume, prepayment provides the incentive to control cost per member by controlling volume without compromising service quality. Controlling volume is the most difficult task to be learned by the provider who is switching from fee-for-service to capitation reimbursement.

With the exception of a few programs that offer only ambulatory care, prepaid plans emphasize the coordinated delivery of inpatient and outpatient care. By giving the health-care provider the financial responsibility for both, savings obtained by achieving lower levels of admissions, lengths of stay, and lower per day hospital costs can be used to provide broader ambulatory coverage such as preventive services, routine office visits, and well-child care. These are services normally not covered by conventional insurance. There is little evidence that providers at risk for only ambulatory care can accomplish the levels of savings comparable to providers at risk for both ambulatory and inpatient care.

In other words, HMOs operating in a competitive marketplace must provide both inpatient and outpatient care economically in order to provide broader benefits than do their competitors and for the same or less cost. Successful prepaid plans that earn a good reputation for quality and price competition in the employer marketplace can also provide high-quality care to Medicaid recipients usually at a rate lower than the fee-for-service system.

Service to Medicaid Recipients in Federally Qualified HMOs

In early 1981 the Health Care Financing Administration and the Public Health Service released the *Report of the Joint HCFA-PHS Task Force on HMO–Medicaid Contracting*. The report strongly endorsed the further promotion of state contracting with federally qualified HMOs. It stated that HMOs "improve beneficiary access to high quality comprehensive health care, save public dollars through the efficient delivery of needed health service to Medicaid beneficiaries and contribute to the containment of Federal and State expenditures through a competitive rather than a regulatory approach."[12]

Historically, Congress, through Title XIII of the Public Health Service Act and the Medicaid provisions of the Social Security Act, has expressed its intent that HMOs serve low-income populations.[12] Nevertheless, as of June 1980 only 23 percent of the prepaid health plans (including federally qualified HMOs) in the country had signed contracts with state Medicaid agencies, and only seventeen states were involved. These contracts covered 270,000 Medicaid beneficiaries, or little more than 1 percent of all beneficiaries.[12]

To most HMOs, economic viability does not depend on serving a Medicaid population, as their success is primarily a function of marketability to the employed population. The Medicaid population does, however, present an additional market to HMOs, and most view service to Medicaid to be an important service to their communities. However, because of the uncertainty of future funding for Medicaid, HMOs should not depend too heavily on Medicaid income.

In many states, Medicaid contracts are difficult to negotiate. The unattractiveness of contract provisions, payment delays, and the difficulties with Medicaid marketing and enrollment present obstacles to furthering HMO participation in Medicaid.

Rate-Setting Issues

There are several attributes of Medicaid contracts that present problems to HMOs. Under increasing pressure to control Medicaid costs, states are often unwilling to negotiate a capitation rate that is sufficient to meet the HMOs actual costs and state-imposed reserve and reinsurance requirements. Establishing prospective capitation payments for HMOs is a major problem for some Medicaid agencies. Many lack skill at rate setting as well as the necessary use and cost data required to set rates. Furthermore, states criticize HMOs for excessive administrative costs and high profits.

When HMOs negotiate rates with state Medicaid agencies, comparisons of HMO costs to those of the fee-for-service sector inevitably occur. While research in Massachusetts, Washington, D.C., and elsewhere point to substantial savings in HMOs, many state officials are still not believers. However, data to settle the argument over HMO rate requests or Medicaid fee-for-service costs are not available.

The implementation of state Medicaid management-information systems offers hope that this situation will improve. However, if state agencies are forced to reimburse physicians and hospitals at low levels due to Medicaid budget constraints, HMOs may have difficulty competing and at the same time serving Medicaid patients. In Pennsylvania, for example, Medicaid reimburses physicians with a fee schedule that is considerably below that of Blue Shield or most other payors. In addition, hospitals claim that reimbursement levels from Medicaid are substantially below their costs. State law requires that HMOs shall not cost Medicaid more than care in other settings. Pennsylvania HMOs may have to reduce their rates below their costs to arrive at levels that are at or under artificially low state costs for Medicaid recipients in the fee-for-service sector. Since many HMOs are small and struggling to attain financial viability, they are not able to enter into a Medicaid contract under these circumstances.

HMOs entering into a Medicaid contract for the first time must do so without the benefit of actual experience upon which to calculate rates. The biggest risk to the HMO is the provision of inpatient hospital care. In the typical HMO-Medicaid contract, approximately 40 percent of the capitation rate is for inpatient hospitalization. An HMO entering into an initial contract not only must establish the hospital capitation with no experience but must also incur the added risk of covering a small first-year enrollment where a few high-cost hospital episodes can send the HMO's costs way above the capitation level and endanger the financial stability of the program.

If the state and the HMO opt for a risk contract, the HMO may attempt to negotiate the following:

A risk-sharing arrangement whereby the state shares losses above budgeted levels of hospitalization and savings for experience below budgeted levels.

A provision whereby the state agrees to cover the cost of or directly underwrite individual stop-loss insurance that will cover the HMO for costs of hospitalization above a certain amount.

A provision whereby the state covers the cost of or directly underwrites risk of insolvency insurance for Medicaid enrollees.

These concepts—risk sharing, reinsurance, and insolvency protection—are highly technical and beyond the normal methods of doing business for state Medicaid agencies. They are critical concepts, however, since Medicaid agencies should be vitally concerned that contracting HMOs are financially sound and adequately protected against insolvency.

Another related issue in rate negotiations is the administrative-cost component of the rate. Typically, administrative costs for smaller HMOs are between 10 and 15 percent of their community rate. Larger HMOs experience less than 10 percent administrative costs. In addition to their normal costs for operating the plan, HMOs must build in additional costs for managing a Medicaid contract. These include special Medicaid-reporting requirements; marketing costs; and costs of membership billing, reconciliation, and membership maintenance. In general, HMOs must add staff, particularly in their marketing and billing departments, to handle the administration of the Medicaid contract, although states are often unwilling to pay for levels of administrative cost to accommodate these added functions.

Although these issues all present problems, none are insurmountable with flexible and openminded negotiations. To protect themselves from some of the high risk of entering into a new Medicaid contract, HMOs may wish to have cost rather than risk contracts for the first two years or so. Both the HMO's ability to gain experience and the state's improved data capabilities through Medicaid management-information systems should provide both parties with more information and therefore more confidence when they sit down to negotiate rates.

Eligibility Determination

The major problem the HMO faces in providing coverage to the Medicaid population is its lack of continuous eligibility, for the status of the poor constantly changes. Once a person is determined to be no longer eligible for benefits, Medicaid funds are no longer available to pay premiums. Some states determine eligibility retroactively. Under these circumstances HMOs may deliver service and then receive no premium payments from the states.

As part of contractual agreements between the HMO and the state, the state should agree to make capitation payments until it has notified the HMO that a beneficiary is no longer eligible. Thus, states should keep a close watch on eligibility and make sure that the HMO is notified on a timely basis. This process is currently so complex and problematic that it is often a source of conflict between the HMO and the state.

From the HMO's perspective, fluctuating eligibility (and thus high member turnover) increases marketing costs and makes it difficult to develop continuous medical-care relationships with a sizeable percentage of their Medicaid enrollment. In situations in which HMOs are not notified that a Medicaid recipient has lost eligibility, the HMO will continue to provide service but may not receive premium payments for months during which services were provided. Particularly in situations in which the HMO is obligated to pay its providers in advance, not receiving premium payments for recipients whom the HMO counted in its membership can represent sizeable losses to the plan.

Inevitably, when states are unable to keep track of eligibility or to notify the HMO on a timely basis, difficulties arise with determining the number of eligible recipients on a month-to-month basis and therefore the total amount of the monthly premium payment due to the HMO by the state. It is not uncommon for HMOs to go month after month in disputes with state agencies regarding large sums of money.

This problem can and does discourage HMOs from serving Medicaid recipients. Several solutions have been previously suggested. In addition to these, under existing federal law, states may guarantee eligibility for a Medicaid eligible enrolled in an HMO for up to six months. Guaranteed eligibility represents an additional cost, but this cost is shared by the federal government. Assuming states are convinced that they save with Medicaid-HMO contracts, they may be willing to incur the additional costs of guaranteed eligibility.

Payment Delays

Late payments by the state has been a major problem for some HMOs. Disputes between the HMO and the state regarding numbers of recipients eligible is a major reason for late payments. In addition, some HMOs have found that payment of rates that have been renegotiated to reflect cost increases and inflation has been delayed by the state because of budgetary considerations. In these situations, states will pay at prenegotiated levels sometimes for long periods until the budget authorities in the state approve payment at the higher negotiated levels. Cash-flow delays and uncertain monthly premium levels are difficult for a young HMO to manage.

Marketing

Marketing and enrollment problems, including the lack of direct access to eligible populations and difficulty convincing Medicaid recipients to give away their Medicaid cards, are often cited by HMOs as major reasons for their lack of interest in enrolling Medicaid beneficiaries.

Unlike employed groups, Medicaid beneficiaries are not identifiable to HMOs for the purpose of marketing because of statutory prohibitions under the Federal Privacy Act concerning the release of beneficiary information. As a result, the HMOs must resort to expensive and administratively complex approaches of marketing to this population, principally the employment of a door-to-door sales force. Door-to-door marketing carries with it the potential for abuse such as that experienced with some Medicaid HMOs in California.

In other ways marketing to Medicaid recipients is different than employer group populations. Medicaid eligibles do not, for example, always obtain broader benefits with the HMO either because the state's Medicaid-benefit package is comprehensive or because the premium rate is insufficient to support extra benefits. Therefore, beneficiaries are likely to be reluctant to give up freedom to seek care from any willing provider where there are no economic or benefit advantages.

Also, some HMOs are reluctant to market actively to Medicaid beneficiaries out of fear of acquiring a "welfare" image. This is of particular concern to new HMOs that are seeking to attract a middle-class enrollment base. HMOs, however, that have not achieved the breakeven enrollment base or that have excess capacity may welcome a Medicaid contract.

Offering Medicaid Required Benefits

In some states Medicaid-benefit requirements are different, and in some cases even broader than, the HMO's own comprehensive benefits package. In Pennsylvania, for example, an HMO with a Medicaid contract must provide dental and pharmacy services in addition to their basic package. Not only must the HMO make these services available but they must have sufficient control over the providers of these services so as to control costs and stay within capitation budgets. HMOs inexperienced with a service such as dental with a potentially high risk may not wish to contract with Medicaid if they must make this service available.

Conclusion

These practical problems should not unduly discourage health organizations from seeking Medicaid contracts. With creative contracts, particularly taking advantage of new provisions under the Medicaid Amendments of 1981 such as guaranteed-eligibility periods and the opportunity to provide financial incentives to recipients to join, there is potential for Medicaid contracts to greatly benefit the state and the HMO.

Many HMOs have provided excellent services to Medicaid recipients and derived the satisfaction of delivering a much-needed service through creative contracting with states. The problems can be extensive but so can the rewards. HMOs have the responsibility, if possible, to venture into this arena for they have the most potential to serve and to reduce costs.

Notes

1. Public Law 97–35 Section, Medicaid Provisions, Omnibus Budget Reconciliation Act of 1981, August 13, 1981.

2. *National HMO Census, 1981*, Office of Health Maintenance Organizations, U.S. Department of Health and Human Services.

3. *Investors Guide to HMOs*, Office of Health Maintenance Organizations, U.S. Department of Health and Human Services, 1982.

4. Harold M. Ting, *Factors Affecting Use of HMOs by Medicaid Program*, ICF Corporation, 1981.

5. N. Fuller and M. Patera, *Report on a Study of Medicaid Utilization of Services in a Prepaid Group Practice Plan* (U.S. Department of Health, Education and Welfare/Social and Rehabilitation Services, Washington, D.C., January 1976).

6. C.R. Gaus, C.B. Cooper, and C. Hirschman, "Contrasts in HMO and Fee-for-Service Performance," *Social Security Bulletin* 39 no. 5 (May 1976): 13–14.

7. T.J. Columbo, D.K. Freeborn, J.P. Mullooly, and V.R. Burnham, "The Effect of Outreach Worker's Education Efforts on Use of Preventive Services by a Poverty Population," Paper Delivered at the American Public Health Association Annual Meeting, Miami (November 1976).

8. C. Colton, R. Neisular, and R.S. Lurie, *Evaluation of a Program to Facilitate the Integration of a Low Income Population Into a Prepaid Group Practice Plan* (Harvard Community Health Plan: Cambridge, July 1976).

9. N. Fuller and M. Patera, 1976.

10. C.R. Gaus, N.A. Fuller, and C. Bohannum, "HMO Evaluation: Utilization Before and After Enrollment," Paper delivered at the American

Public Health Association Annual Meeting, Atlantic City, N.J., November 1972.

11. Harold S. Luft, *Health Maintenance Organizations: Dimensions of Performance*, chap. 13, Health Policy Program, University of California, San Franciso (New York: Wiley, 1981).

12. *Report of the Joint HCFA–PHS Task Force on HMO-Medicaid Contracting* U.S. Department of Health and Human Services, December 1980.

**Part V
Current Research Findings**

13 Medical and Socioeconomic Case Mix in Outpatient Departments

Joanna Lion and
Judith LaVor Williams

Medical and socioeconomic case-mix differences have long been thought to be a major reason for the cost differential between a visit to a hospital OPD and to a private physician's office. Many have argued that teaching-hospital OPDs in particular see patients who are medically sicker and who have more social problems. The combination of these factors is assumed to explain the higher costs of OPD visits.

This chapter examines these two issues. First, it examines the available evidence for medical-case-mix differences between hospital OPDs and private practices using a large-scale, nationwide data set developed in the late 1970s. It then examines data from a recent survey conducted in three Boston teaching-hospital OPDs, looking first at medical case mix within these OPDs and then turning to findings about socioeconomic case mix in these settings. It then looks at use of OPD resources by patients with and without social problems.

The large-scale nationwide data set was developed by the University of Southern California, which conducted a survey using physicians sampled from the American Medical Association Directory of all practicing physicians across the country and on a specialty-specific basis for twenty-four specialties. Findings have been reported elsewhere for four major specialties—internal medicine, pediatrics, family practice, and general practice.[1,2] Much to our surprise, we found that medical-case-mix differences appeared to be relatively minor, when hospital-based residents or salaried staff were compared with private practitioners. The next section of this paper summarizes findings of this work.

Several important questions arose as a result of these findings. One was whether the 10,737 OPD visits reported to the four specialties in the USC-Mendenhall study were representative of large urban teaching-hospital OPDs. In some ways these visits obviously were not since only 41 percent of the 92 million hospital OPD visits in the country take place in teaching

This research has been supported by the Robert Wood Johnson Foundation, Grant 5180, and by the Health Care Financing Administration, Grant 18–P/97905.

161

hospitals of more than four hundred beds (American Hospital Association, unpublished data).

On the other hand, it is quite possible that hospital OPD visits do not differ much in their complexity between inner-city teaching-hospital OPDs and others when the four specialties just mentioned are considered. To test this hypothesis, we conducted a study in three large teaching hospitals in Boston using a two-week sample of visits to their ambulatory-care units. These findings are summarized in the second section of this chapter.

A second question concerns whether medical case mix—measured by such things as primary and secondary diagnoses and the physician's assessment of how severe, complex, and urgent the visits are—is really an adequate measure of the complexity of the patients seen. A frequent argument is that the patients seen in hospital OPDs are more difficult to treat because they have more social and economic problems than patients seen in other settings.

Since the USC-Mendenhall data set had no information on social problems, we used our original data-collection effort in the three Boston hospitals to specifically address this issue. The final portion of this chapter describes early findings from this study. It should be noted that previous researchers have established that patients seen in inner-city hospital OPDs are indeed more beset with social, psychological, and economic problems.[3,4]

Cugliani substantiates large socioeconomic differences between patients seen in New York City OPDs and residents of New York City. She indicates that patients seen in the OPD also are sicker on self-reported measures than patients seen by private practitioners but offers only anecdotal evidence in support of her contention. A number of small-scale studies indicate that patients seen in hospital OPDs are of lower socioeconomic status than those seen in private practice.[5,6,7] These patients also appear to have a substantial number of psychosocial problems. For example, 36 percent of an OPD pediatric sample presented with psychosocial problems *only* and an additional 52 percent with psychosocial problems in addition to physical ones.[8]

Given this heavier social-problem mix in hospital OPDs, one must address the question of whether patients with these problems actually use more hospital OPD resources than patients without. This chapter leaves many issues unsettled since much of the data is based on preliminary analysis. Nevertheless, the data presented here represent a new body of knowledge about hospital OPDs. These data tend to support our earlier findings that the cost differential between hospital OPDs and private practice *cannot* be attributed primarily to the different types of patients served.

Medical-Case-Mix Differences between OPDs
and Private Practice

Using two different techniques, a case-mix difference of at most 5 to 15
percent can be demonstrated between hospital OPDs and patients of physicians in private practice, at least as far as patients of primary-care specialists
are concerned. Table 13–1 summarizes these findings using an ambulatory-
visit group methodology that was developed at Yale and is similar in concept
and effect to diagnostic-related groups (DRGs) for inpatients.

The USC-Mendenhall data set samples physicians by specialty. The vast
majority of the visits reported by each group of specialists were to physicians

Table 13–1
Comparison of Case Mix by Specialty, with Percent Differences,
Using Autogrouping

Specialty and Type of Practice	Time in Minutes			Percent More Complex[a]	Percent Less Efficient[a]
	Actual Length of Encounter	Expected Length of Encounter	Mean for Specialty		
Private Practice					
Internal medicine	15.10	15.33	15.59	—	—
Pediatrics	9.18	9.43	9.59	—	—
Family practice	9.07	9.38	9.48	—	—
General practice	9.06	9.36	9.39	0.5	—
Salaried Hospital Staff					
Internal medicine	18.08	16.18	15.59	5.6	13.4
Pediatrics	12.00	10.79	9.59	15.0	14.2
Family practice	9.79	9.57	9.48	2.0	5.5
General practice	10.50	9.31	9.39	—	16.7
Residents					
Internal medicine	19.32	17.32	15.59	13.0	13.2
Pediatrics	13.18	10.67	9.59	12.9	27.3
Family practice	13.01	10.21	9.48	9.1	31.3
General practice	12.38	9.50	9.39	1.8	34.3

Source: USC-Mendenhall data on 84,590 ambulatory-patient visits run through the AVG
program developed by Yale.

Note: *Autogrouping* is a method of explaining as much variance in physician time as possible
by assigning patients to a series of groups based on their demographic and medical characteristics. It was developed at Yale and is similar to inpatient diagnostically related groups (DRGs)
in its structure.

[a]Complexity is obtained by dividing column 2 by column 3; efficiency is obtained by dividing
column 1 by column 2. The resulting ratios are converted to percents by standardizing the
lowest figure in the group at unity (1.000).

in private practice. Of the 84,590 visits included in table 13–1, 13 percent were to hospital OPDs. For more detailed information on how the USC-Mendenhall data set was developed, including the log-diary approach by which the sampled physicians recorded data on all patient visits for a three-day period, a number of previous publications are available.[9,10,11]

For the autogrouping analysis producing table 13–1, all visits are divided into the final groups developed at Yale and then are redistributed into the three practice settings under consideration. This analysis produces the actual mean length of encounter for each practice setting (19.32 minutes for internal-medicine residents, for example) compared with internists as a whole (15.59).

The data for each type of practice setting are then rerun through the program and are recalculated based on the percent of visits for that type of practice in each of the final groups multiplied by the mean time it takes for all patients in the group to be seen. This figure is the expected length of encounter. In other words, the expected length of encounter was calculated by determining for each type of practice what proportion of their patients was in each of the final groups and then multiplying that proportion by the mean encounter time for the group. For residents, the figure was 17.32 minutes. The calculation indicates that residents should be taking only 17.32 minutes to see their particular mix of patients compared to the 19.32 minutes they are actually taking. In fact, both types of OPD physicians spent significantly more time with their patients than indicated if they were adhering to the mean times established for all patients for each of the groups.

The formal relationship for the time residents take to treat their patients is shown by the ratio of actual time to expected time, which is 1.115, indicating that residents are taking 11.5 percent longer to treat their patients than indicated by their case mix. More important for the purposes of this discussion, the expected length of encounter for residents is longer than the group average length of encounter, giving a ratio of 1.111. This figure indicates that residents in internal medicine actually have a case mix 11 percent sicker than the average and about 13 percent sicker than internists in private practice, who have an expected length of encounter slightly less than the group average and a case-mix ratio of 0.983. These figures were then converted to a base that standardizes the lowest ratio at unity for each analysis.

For seven of the eight comparisons possible, patients seen in the OPD were both more complex to treat and took longer to treat, even considering their complexity, than patients in private practice. In the one aberrant case, general-practice complexity, the differences were very small across sites. The two specialty primary practices, internal medicine and pediatrics, showed greater differences, again consistent with anecdotal evidence.

Medical Case Mix in Teaching-Hospital OPDs

Because of the implications for reimbursement policy of the finding that little case-mix difference exists, we are still working with our data to tease out possible alternative explanations and to check as much as possible the validity of the findings. One of the major criticisms of our findings is that large inner-city OPDs have much sicker patients than OPDs in general. Since the USC-Mendenhall study's unit for sampling was a sample of physicians throughout the country, their data are representative of OPDs in general. It is not possible to break out teaching-hospital OPDs from USC-Mendenhall, leading us to undertake a separate study to examine the possibility that large teaching hospitals are different in their OPD-patient mix.

The hospitals in whose primary-care clinics we conducted our study are teaching hospitals located in the city of Boston. Two, Beth Israel (BIAC) and New England Medical Center (NEMC), are private, nonprofit hospitals, and the third, Boston City Hospital (BCH), is owned and operated by the city. All are of approximately the same size on the inpatient side, having about 450 beds. The two voluntary hospitals have about 25,000 visits per year in their primary-care and walk-in clinics combined, excluding Ob-Gyn and pediatrics, and the municipal hospital sees about 31,000. The types of patients seen differ somewhat among the OPDs and between the walk-in and appointment clinics.

All the hospitals have tried to structure their primary-care clinics to varying degrees along group-practice lines, emphasizing continuity of care. They also, however, maintain staff to see walk-in patients, who are either diverted from the emergency department or have no regular physician or have other reasons for seeking this type of care. We have no data on the Beth Israel walk-in clinic (BIAC). Data from the NEMC walk-in clinic is incomplete and has been omitted from the analysis in this chapter. Table 13–2 shows the response rates for the three hospitals.

Table 13–2
Number of Visits and Completion Rates, Three Boston Hospital Outpatient Departments

Completion Rate	BIAC	BCH Appointments	BCH Walk-Ins	NEMC	All Visits
Number of visits in two-week period	874	678	669	666	2,887
Number of usable questionnaires	435	625	626	651	2,337
Completion rate	49.8%	92.2%	93.6%	97.8%	81.0%

It should be remembered that the USC-Mendenhall data shown in this chapter are based on visits across the ambulatory-care spectrum, with only 13 percent of the visits being to internists and internal-medicine residents in the OPD. An even more meaningful comparison would entail using only visits to the OPD; however, this is not possible using existing data. Another difference that makes the comparison less than ideal is that the Mendenhall data set is based on a sample of physician practices regardless of setting, while our study is based on patients seen by providers in specific settings. Thus our data includes patients of nurse practitioners and, in one clinic, patients seen by social workers.

Finally, since the Mendenhall data were sampled by specialty, we had to choose between internal medicine and family practice as the most logical comparison with our study. It turns out that the vast majority of physicians seeing patients in the three urban-hospital clinics we studied are internists or internal-medicine subspecialists. This, plus the fact that the patients seen in all three primary-care clinics are limited to adults who do not have pregnancy as their primary diagnosis, persuaded us to compare with the USC-Mendenhall internal-medicine data.

The tables in this chapter are based on 2,337 visits to primary-care and walk-in clinics in three Boston teaching hospitals; 819 to staff physicians, mostly internists; 1,085 to residents, mostly in internal medicine; 396 to nurse practitioners; and 37 to social workers. The municipal hospital used a preponderance of residents, mostly in their walk-in clinic, and the two private hospitals a preponderance of salaried staff physicians. Table 13–3 compares data from the primary-care clinics of the three urban hospitals we have studied to all ambulatory visits in the USC-Mendenhall data set.

Our tentative conclusion is that the patients of urban-hospital primary-care units do not look too different in their leading diagnoses from the patients of physicians in private practice. Hypertension is the leading diagnosis in all three settings, with diabetes, anxiety and depression, and osteoarthritis also high on the list. Medical exams are less prominent for the inner-city OPDs, but even here medical exam as a reason for visit is fourth on the list for the municipal hospital. This is partly because of its function in providing physical examinations for employment or transportation passes, as well as for residents of nursing homes and group homes for the mentally retarded. One of the private-hospital OPDs had an unusually large number of visits for emotional problems as the primary diagnosis, possibly because of the social workers who see patients there. The municipal hospital, on the other hand, has alcoholism in its top ten diagnoses.

Another issue is whether case mix varies by type of clinic. While this seems self-evident for tertiary clinics compared with primary-care clinics, it is less obvious that the adult-medicine primary-care clinic actually consists of two clinics, a regular appointment clinic and a walk-in clinic designed to

Table 13–3
Comparison of USC-Mendenhall Leading Diagnoses for Ambulatory Care with Primary Diagnoses in Three Large Boston Teaching Hospitals

Diagnosis	USC-Mendenhall[a]		BIAC		BCH		NEMC		All	
Hypertension	10.4%	(1)	22.1%	(1)	17.6%	(1)	18.9%	(1)	18.8	(1)
Chronic ischemic heart disease	6.6	(2)	3.5	(5)	0.6		4.3	(3)	2.2	(5)
Medical exam	6.4	(3)	1.2		2.7	(4)	1.2		2.0	(9)
Diabetes	5.0	(4)	7.8	(2)	7.8	(2)	4.1	(4)	6.8	(2)
Acute upper-respiratory infection	3.3	(5)			1.4		0.3		0.9	
Neuroses	2.6	(6)	7.8	(2)	2.2	(7)	4.6	(2)	3.9	(3)
Osteoarthritis	2.0	(7)	4.6	(4)	3.2	(3)	2.2	(7)	3.2	(4)
Symptomatic heart disease	1.7	(8)	2.1	(7)	1.5		3.5	(5)	2.2	(5)
Influenza	1.5	(9)			0.2				0.1	
Obesity	1.6	(10)	0.5		0.7		1.7	(9)	0.9	
Angina			2.1	(7)	0.5				0.6	
Chronic obstructive pulmonary disease			1.8	(7)	1.3		3.1	(6)	1.9	(10)
Asthma			2.8	(6)	2.4	(6)	1.2		2.1	(8)
Personality disorders			2.1	(7)	0.1				0.4	
Convulsive disorder			2.1	(7)			1.4	(10)	0.8	
Alcoholism			1.2		2.0	(8)	0.6		1.5	
Abdominal pain			0.9		1.7	(10)	0.9		1.3	
Urinary-tract infection			0.5		2.6	(5)	1.8	(8)	2.0	(7)
Myalgia, neuralgia, pain in limbs			0.9		1.8	(9)	0.9		1.4	
Back pain, disorders			0.9		0.1		1.4	(10)	0.6	
Cumulative percent accounted for by top ten diagnoses	41.1		55.4		44.0		45.6		45.5	

Note: Based on ICD-8 and ICD-9-CM matched for these diagnoses to three digits. Numbers in parentheses are the rank order of diagnoses.
[a]Based on 19,764 ambulatory visits to internists in all settings.

divert nonemergency patients away from the emergency room. Although both types of clinics—and their patients—are focused on primary care, they differ substantially in a number of respects. Thus we are treating the walk-in and appointment patients as two separate groups for part of our analysis.

Table 13–4 compares the top ten diagnoses of the two primary-care patient groups at BCH. Several points are immediately obvious from the table:

1. The walk-in patients exhibit a greater variety of illness than the appointment patients; the top ten diagnoses account for only about 30 percent of all walk-in visits compared with 60 percent of the appointments.

Table 13–4

Comparison of Leading Diagnoses in Appointment and Walk-In Ambulatory-Care Clinics in a Municipal Teaching Hospital

ICD-9 Code	Primary Diagnosis	BCH Appointments		BCH Walk-In	
(401)	Hypertension	28.1%	(1)	7.3%	(1)
(250)	Diabetes	13.6	(2)	2.1	(9)
(493)	Asthma	3.5	(3)	1.3	
(300,311)	Neuroses	2.8	(4)	1.6	
(715-6)	Osteoarthritis	2.6	(5)	3.8	(4)
(427-8)	Symptomatic heart disease	2.4	(6)	.5	
(496)	Chronic obstructive pulmonary disease	2.2	(7)	.5	
(303)	Alcoholism	1.9	(8)	2.2	(8)
(571)	Alcoholic liver damage	1.3	(9)		
(533)	Peptic ulcer	1.3	(9)	.9	
(780)	Convulsive disorders, dizziness	1.3	(9)	1.8	
(599)	Urinary-tract infection			4.8	(2)
(729)	Myalgia, neuralgia, pain in limbs			3.0	(5)
(079)	Viral infection			2.6	(6)
(V68,V70)	Medical exam			4.6	(3)
(465)	Acute upper-respiratory infection			2.4	(7)
(789)	Abdominal pain			2.1	(9)
	Cumulative percent accounted for by top ten diagnoses	59.7		30.3	

2. The case mix of the appointment patient group of BCH resembles that of the private appointment clinics (see table 13–3).
3. Minor infections, such as upper-respiratory infections, and symptoms figure much more heavily in the top diagnoses of the walk-in patients. (It takes one to three weeks to get an appointment in the OPD, which would explain why minor acute conditions, which are self-limiting, appear only among the walk-in patients.)
4. A higher proportion of the appointment patients have chronic diagnoses common to middle age and old age. As might be expected, the appointment patients as a group are considerably older than the walk-ins.

Social Problems Reported in OPDs

This section describes the socioeconomic case mix of the three urban teaching-hospital OPDs in which we collected data. The major socioeconomic variables included in our questionnaire were an openended question about the presence and types of social problems for each patient, race, third-party payer, and language problems, including need for an interpreter. In addition, we expanded on the USC-Mendenhall questionnaire by adding time for professional practitioners other than physicians. Thus nurse practitioners were considered providers, and time was also collected for preceptors, consultants, interpreters, and social workers.

Table 13–5 provides some basic sociodemographic data for the visits to the three primary-care clinics studied. The overall percentage of minorities and of patients sixty-five and over is considerably higher than for the Boston population as a whole. Blacks account for 22.4 percent of Boston's population but 45.6 percent of our total patient visits. Hispanics are underrepresented in two of the three facilities: Boston's Hispanic population is 6.4 percent, roughly the same as that of Boston City Hospital's sample. The proportion of visits by elderly patients is, at 26.6 percent, more than twice that of the Boston population as a whole where 12.7 percent is over sixty-five.[12] Older people, of course, have more visits than younger ones, so it is less than ideal to compare a data base with visits as the unit of observation with population data.

Economic problems, here indicated by the proportion of visits by patients on Medicaid or with no third-party payer, also exceed the proportion in the population as a whole. Over half the visits overall fit into this category, while only 16 percent of Boston's population is on Medicaid; nationally only about 10 percent of all patients have no third-party coverage.

The types of social problems reported for patients in the three primary-care clinics are presented in table 13–6. The sixteen variables listed were developed from write-ins of social problems by the providers.

Table 13–5
Demographic Data for Visits to the Three Boston Teaching-Hospital Primary-Care Clinics

Demographic Data for Visits	BIAC Appointments[a]	BCH Appointments	BCH Walk-In	NEMC Appointments	All Visits
Percent under thirty	11.3	7.2	36.3	9.6	16.4
Percent over sixty-five	33.6	30.2	11.2	33.0	26.6
Percent black	35.2	62.9	70.1	12.4	45.6
Percent Hispanic[b]	0.7	6.7	6.1	2.3	4.2
Percent Oriental	1.4	0.5	1.3	4.3	1.9
Percent on Medicaid[c]	38.6	36.5	21.9	25.4	28.4
Percent with *no* third-party payer[d]	6.7	26.1	47.8	7.4	23.7

[a]BIAC was actually sampled on a 50-percent basis and surveyed for one month.

[b]Blacks of Hispanic origin are not double-counted but are coded under black rather than Hispanic.

[c]Includes Medicaid as only payer and Medicaid backing up Medicare.

[d]Virtually all these patients are nonpaying. Included are self-pay, part-pay, no-pay, and general-relief patients. At present general relief does not cover outpatient care in Massachusetts.

Table 13-6
Social Problems Encountered in Three Boston Outpatient Departments
(percent of visits)

Classification of Social Problems	Mentioned as Social Problem[a]			Mentioned as Medical Problem Only[b]			Mentioned as Either
	BIAC	BCH	NEMC	BIAC	BCH	NEMC	All Hospitals
Minor Problem							
Anxiety	24.4	3.1	8.5	0.5	0.2	0.3	8.8
Depression	20.0	6.0	10.0	7.6	3.3	5.7	15.7
Minor psychological	7.1	8.7	8.2	6.7	3.2	4.1	12.3
Ex-alcoholic	3.4	1.2	1.5				1.5
Obesity	0.9	1.6	1.4	12.4	9.6	10.6	12.0
Medical noncompliance	2.3	4.0	3.1				3.1
Difficulty being understood[c]	4.9	5.8	1.7				4.5
Moderate Problem							
Family problems	26.0	10.5	13.6		0.1	0.1	13.7
Financial problems	19.1	16.4	14.9		0.1	0.0	14.9
Living/situational problems	2.5	5.3	5.2			0.1	5.3
Housing problems	0.2	2.9	2.1		0.1		2.1
Major Problem							
Alcoholism	5.0	5.7	5.1	0.2	2.2	2.4	7.5
Drug abuse	2.3	2.5	2.1	0.9	1.7	1.4	3.5
Mental retardation	1.1	0.8	0.9	0.2	0.3	0.3	1.2
Physical disability	7.8	3.5	4.0	1.6	2.1	2.2	6.2
Major psychiatric	2.3	1.4	1.8	2.5	2.8	2.3	4.1
Needs an interpreter[c]	6.9	6.3	4.0				5.7

[a]Up to three social problems per patient could be coded so that the sum of these percents is greater than the percent of patients with a social problem
[b]Not mentioned as a social problem but given as a primary or secondary diagnosis using ICD-9-CM.
[c]These were originally both part of a social problem called "language difficulties."

During our preliminary analysis of the data, we reduced the number of social problems by grouping them under broader variables and looked also at whether what we defined as social problems were instead being considered as a medical diagnosis by some providers. This method added slightly to the number of people with social problems, though only one problem, obesity, was overwhelmingly mentioned as a diagnosis. Psychological problems such as depression and other "minor" and major problems were heavily listed as diagnoses rather than social problems. Senility and brain damage were the major psychological problems most apt to be considered as a medical diagnosis.

A definition of social problem which includes patients listed as having that problem either as a diagnosis or as a social problem indicates that 61.8 percent of the patients seen in Boston hospital OPDs had at least one social problem. Interestingly, one of the private hospitals had a much higher percentage of patients with reported social problems than did the municipal hospital. This finding may be the result of perceived relative deprivation in the case of financial problems and to the presence of social workers as part of the primary-care clinic. Patients with anxiety and depression may be referred to the mental-health clinics of the other two hospitals.

The division into patients with minor, moderate, and major social problems reveals that the municipal-hospital patients were thought to have more serious problems. As can be seen in table 13–7, the breakdown by seriousness of the problems splits almost evenly for BIAC, while at the city hospital the more serious problems predominate. The question to be addressed in further analysis is whether these severity gradations bear any relation to time and resources used to treat the patients. This issue is further explored in the next section.

One measure that might bear on resource use is the physician's estimate of how difficult the patient is to assess and treat, considering all of his problems. This measure is called "complexity" and was developed by the USC-Mendenhall staff from the American Medical Association current procedural terminology (CPT) scale.

Patients with complexity ratings of 4 and 5 on a scale of 5 are examined in table 13–8. These rankings are based on the USC-Mendenhall definitions of extended and comprehensive encounters demanding unusual time and skill. Medical diagnosis is not controlled for in table 13–8 but is assumed to distribute at random among the people with social problems.

Only three of the social problems did not contribute to an overall complexity in handling the patient that was greater than the average for patients without a social problem. One of these social problems—obesity—was also the only one that was overwhelmingly mentioned as a medical rather than a social problem. One of the other social problems—difficulties with language, including need for an interpreter or other language difficulty—probably does not make the patient more complex to handle but does require additional time. The third problem that did not appear to contribute to complexity was economic. The most complex cases to treat appear to be drug abusers (the drug usually mentioned is heroin); ex-alcoholics; and the homeless (many of them street people, temporary-

Table 13–7
Percent of Patients with Social Problems, by Severity of Problem

	Percent of Patients with Problems			
Severity of Problem	*BIAC*	*BCH*	*NEMC*	*All OPDs*
No social problem	25.3	41.7	40.1	38.2
Minor	21.6	13.7	21.7	17.4
Moderate	27.1	17.6	18.3	19.6
Major	26.0	27.0	20.0	24.9

Table 13–8
Percent of Visits Where Overall Care Was Considered
More Complex than Average, Ranked by Type of Social
Problem for All Three Hospitals Combined

Social Problem	Percent with Very or Extremely Complex Care	Number of Cases with the Problem[a]
Drug abuse	39.5	81
Ex-alcoholic	38.2	34
Homeless	31.2	48
Family problems	29.2	319
Mentally retarded	28.6	28
Minor psychological problems	28.6	287
Major psychiatric problems	28.4	95
Blind, deaf, physically disabled	26.4	144
Living problems	25.0	124
Depression	25.0	368
Alcoholic	25.0	176
Anxiety	24.6	207
Medical noncompliance	23.6	72
Economic problem	21.1	74
Needs interpreter	20.9	134
Other language difficulty	20.2	104
Obesity	17.8	281
Patients with a social problem	25.1	1445
Patients without a social problem	22.1	892
All patients combined	23.9	2337

Note: These data include all practitioners.

[a]This adds up to more than the total since each case can have up to three problems coded and could conceivably have more than three social problems when medical diagnosis is used as well.

shelter residents, and alcoholics). Since an individual may have more than a single social problem recorded, many fall into more than one category.

In order to address this problem, mutually exclusive categories of social problems were created, with a person's being assigned to the category of his most severe problem. A modified Delphi technique was used to develop the categories. The problems falling into each category have already been shown in table 13–6. When complexity is evaluated for minor, moderate, and severe social problems, it increases in small steps in a logical progression for all hospitals combined. Patients with no social problem were considered more complex than average to treat 22.1 percent of the time, compared to 22.4 percent with minor, 25.4 percent with moderate, and 26.7 percent with severe social problems.

Does Social Case Mix Affect Patient-Encounter Time?

We have already seen that patients with social problems are considered more complex to treat than those without and that patients with the "most serious" problems (determined subjectively a priori) are considered to be more complex to treat than those with "minor" problems. Since the complexity measure was developed from American Medical Association CPT coding, which is intended as a rough measure of physician time for billing purposes, it might be expected that patients with social problems use more time. Since it could also be argued that these patients might have *medical* problems that are more complex than average, we have standardized for diagnosis by comparing physician ratings of complexity and physician time used for people with and without social problems for the top ten diagnoses.

Table 13–9 shows these results. Several points are immediately obvious:

1. Patients with a social problem use about 8 percent more physician time overall before diagnosis is considered.
2. Physicians consider patients with a social problem harder than average

Table 13–9
Physician Time Use by Patient Visits with and without Social Problems, Standardized by Diagnosis

Primary Diagnosis	Percent with Social Problem	Percent with More than Average Complexity		Mean Minutes	
		With a Social Problem	Without a Social Problem	With a Social Problem	Without a Social Problem
Hypertension	57.7	17.1	19.7	22.0	23.2
Diabetes	64.4	27.7	27.8	26.4	22.0
Anxiety and depression	100.0	29.9		26.7	
Osteoarthritis	53.6	32.4	37.5	25.8	25.6
Chronic ischemic heart disease	66.7	32.1	21.4	25.5	28.1
Symptomatic heart disease	56.1	21.7	16.7	24.2	25.7
Urinary-tract infection	44.7	33.3	19.2	28.1	27.0
Asthma	58.5	16.7	5.9	26.8	19.4
Medical examination	29.2	0	17.7	29.8	17.0
Chronic obstructive pulmonary disease	70.0	14.3	0	29.6	25.1
All patients, all diagnoses	57.7	27.5	23.7	25.8	23.8

Note: Data based on 1,943 encounters in which a physician was seen.

to treat 27.5 percent of the time compared with 23.7 percent of the time for patients without a social problem.

3. Of the top ten diagnoses, six require more physician time to treat when the patient has a social problem, three require less time, and one— neuroses— is limited by definition to patients with a social problem.
4. Of the six diagnoses where social problems complicate the treatment, two diagnoses—medical examinations and asthma—are especially affected. A person with a social problem undergoing a medical examination uses 75 percent more physician time; a person with asthma, 38 percent more.

There is some indication that, were our cell sizes large enough to also standardize for age, the young would receive more physician time than the old regardless of social problems. One study that reran USC-Mendenhall data has shown that, when diagnosis is standardized for, patients over sixty-five receive fewer minutes of physician time than patients forty-five to sixty-four. The assumption was that physicians may be less interested in treating older patients, that is, that old age can be considered a social problem or at least a stigma.[13]

There is, of course, the possibility that patients with social problems are seen disproportionately by nurse practitioners, social workers, and residents, rather than being seen by highly paid staff physicians. If this is the case, the finding that patients with social problems use 8 percent more physician time could be negated by a finding that when provider time is weighted, this difference does not hold up.

Table 13–10 bears on this issue. When *all* provider time is considered, with salaried staff physicians weighted at unity, nurse practitioners at .44, social workers at .40, residents at .35, and interpreters and other direct-service personnel at .30, based on the relationship of salaries, the resources used by patients with social problems *increase* fairly dramatically:

1. Patients with a social problem use 25 percent *more* provider time overall before diagnosis is considered, indicating either that they are more apt to be seen by salaried staff physicians (or that these physicians are more apt to recognize and record social problems); that they are apt to have more than one practitioner see them during the same visit; or they are seen for longer periods by nurses and social workers, cancelling out the savings in using these lower-level practitioners.
2. Of the top ten diagnoses, seven used more weighted provider time when the patient had a social problem.
3. Diagnoses showing the most extreme difference are again medical examinations (62.2 percent more provider time) and asthma (50.0 percent), followed by Chronic Obstructive Pulmonary Disease (45.9 per-

Table 13–10
Provider Time Use by Patient Visits with and without Social Problems, Standardized by Diagnosis

Primary Diagnosis	Percent with Social Problem	Percent with More than Average Complexity		Mean Standardized Minutes	
		With a Social Problem	Without a Social Problem	With a Social Problem	Without a Social Problem
Hypertension	63.4	14.3	17.3	14.6	14.5
Diabetes	71.1	17.7	21.7	15.0	11.2
Neuroses	100.0	31.5	—	21.1	—
Osteoarthritis	54.1	30.0	35.3	20.0	14.2
Chronic ischemic heart disease	72.0	27.8	21.4	21.0	21.1
Symptomatic heart disease	62.0	25.8	15.8	19.2	17.5
Urinary-tract infection	43.8	33.3	18.5	18.6	12.8
Asthma	62.0	12.9	5.3	15.9	10.6
Medical examination	33.3	11.1	16.7	15.9	9.8
Chronic obstructive pulmonary disease	71.1	12.5	0	20.0	13.7
All patients, all diagnoses	61.8	25.1	22.1	17.4	14.0

Note: Data based on 2,337 encounters including physicians, nurse practitioners, social workers, LPNs, interpreters, and any other direct-care staff seeing the patient. Physicians are subdivided into salaried staff physicians and residents, with residents' time weighted to reflect their salaries in the same way that nonphysician time is.

cent), urinary-tract infection (45.3 percent), and osteoarthritis (40.8 percent).

4. Hypertension, far and away the leading diagnosis, shows virtually no difference in time using either of these methods.

An alternative explanation of how social problems affect provider time is that perceptions of social problems may differ among types of providers. Nurse practitioners, for example, either by training or experience, may be more likely to view something as a social problem than are residents or staff physicians.

Table 13–11 indicates that the physician time in the three Boston OPDs is considerably higher than the time spent with patients for internists in all practice settings regardless of diagnosis. This is consistent with previous findings that physicians practicing in OPDs tend to take longer to see the same medical case mix.

The magnitude of the difference is also somewhat higher than might have been expected when comparing OPD-based salaried staff physicians (18.1 minutes) or residents (19.3 minutes) with the OPD mean time per

Table 13–11
Comparison of USC-Mendenhall and Boston Hospital Outpatient
Department Data for Visit Time by Diagnosis

	Mean Time in Minutes	
Primary Diagnosis	USC Mendenhall	Boston OPDs[a]
Hypertension	16.4	22.5
Diabetes	18.4	24.8
Neuroses	20.6	26.7
Osteoarthritis	19.2	25.7
Urinary-tract infection	[b]	27.5
Chronic ischemic heart disease	19.3	26.4
Symptomatic heart disease	21.8	24.9
Asthma	18.2	23.7
Medical exam[c]	26.9	20.8
Chronic obstructive pulmonary disease	19.5	28.3
All patients	15.6	24.9

[a]Nurse practitioners and social workers excluded.

[b]Not available for USC-Mendenhall.

[c]This reversal of direction is almost certainly due to full medical examinations in the USC-Mendenhall data set being compared to walk-in examinations for specific purposes such as bus passes and halfway house admission in the Boston teaching hospitals.

patient in Boston, which is 24.9 minutes. While a sicker medical case mix cannot be entirely ruled out in accounting for most of this difference between all OPDs and the three we examined in the Boston area, preceding comparisons in this paper make this somewhat unlikely. Another possible explanation is the heavy teaching-time component in the Boston hospitals, but this must be investigated in more detail. Further studies should also be undertaken by other investigators to substantiate or disprove the effects of social-case-mix differences shown here.

Conclusions

Our conclusions from all the data we amassed are that, whatever the reasons for the large differential in hospital OPD costs compared to those for a visit in private practice, they cannot be primarily attributed to either medical- or social-case-mix differences.

Assuming that the diagnoses are randomly distributed, only about two minutes or about 8 percent of additional physician time appears to be attributable to the presence of a social problem. Since not all patients have a social problem, the overall effect in a hospital OPD of a 61.8-percent rate of social problems compared with an assumed 10-percent rate in private practice will be on the order of about 4 percent additional physician time required. We have already seen in the first section of this paper that the difference in medical case mix is at most about 10 percent for internists, leading to a sum of less than a 15-percent differential in physician time in favor of OPDs even when medical- and social-case-mix differences are combined.

If the provider time adjustment is made, which allows for including the work of nurse practitioners and social workers and the downweighting of residents compared to salaried staff physicians, patients with social problems require about 25 percent more provider time. This gives a 12.5 percent differential in favor of hospital OPDs.

Assuming an additive rather than interactive effect with medical case mix, we could expect at very most 30 percent more direct-health-care personnel resources used in the OPD compared with private practice in order to handle the increased medical and social problems combined. Since direct-health-care personnel account for about half of all OPD costs, this would translate into a maximum of 15 percent more in absolute terms. This is far less than the very large differential in cost per visit usually observed between OPDs and private practice.

In short, it appears that hospitals must base their case for differential reimbursement primarily on other issues raised in this book, such as providing access to the indigent, higher capital requirements, higher teaching and personnel costs, or other factors. Roughly a fifth of the cost differential—no small amount but far less than has been previously supposed—is found to be due to either medical or social case mix using the most optimistic assumptions. Therefore, although further study is needed, it is apparent that case mix is not the major reason for the differences in costs among settings.

Notes

1. Joanna Lion, "Commentaries: Case Mix Differences Among Ambulatory Patients Seen by Internists in Various Settings," *Health Services Research* 16 (Winter 1981): 4.

2. Joanna Lion and Stuart Altman, "Case-Mix Differences Between Hospital Outpatient Departments and Private Practice," *Health Care Financing Review* 4 (fall 1982): 1.

3. Anne Cugliani, "Patterns of Hospital Based Ambulatory Care," *Social Science & Medicine* 12 (1978).

4. Diana Dutton, "Patterns of Ambulatory Health Care in Five Different Delivery Systems," *Medical Care* XVII, (no. 3) (March 1979).

5. R.E.M. Lees, R. Steele, and R.A. Spasoff, "Primary Care for Non-Traumatic Illness at the Emergency Department and the Family Physician's Office," *Canadian Medical Association Journal*, February 1976.

6. P. Rudd and A.C. Carrier, "Patients of Internists in Hospital Outpatient Departments and in Private Practice," *Canadian Medical Association Journal* 119.8 (October 21, 1978): 891–895.

7. K. Vincent Rudnick, Walter O. Spitzer, and John Pierce, "Comparison of a Private Family Practice and a University Teaching Practice," *Journal of Medical Education* 51, May 1976.

8. Raymond S. Duff, Daniel S. Rowe, and Frederic P. Anderson, "Patient Care and Student Learning in a Pediatric Clinic," *Pediatrics* 50 (1972): 839.

9. Robert C. Mendenhall, Roger A. Girard, and Stephen Abrahamson, "A National Study of Medical and Surgical Specialties: I. Background, Purpose, and Methodology," *Journal of the American Medical Association* 240, no. 9 (September 1, 1978).

10. Robert C. Mendenhall, John S. Lloyd, Paul Repicky, Joanne R. Monson, Roger A. Girard, and Stephen Abrahamson, "A National Study of Medical and Surgical Specialties: II. Description of the Survey Instrument," *Journal of the American Medical Association* 240, no. 11 (September 8, 1978).

11. Linda H. Aiken, Charles E. Lewis, John Craig, Robert C. Mendenhall, Robert J. Blendon, and David E. Rogers, "The Contribution of Specialists to the Delivery of Primary Care: A New Perspective," *New England Journal of Medicine* 300, no. 24 (June 14, 1981).

12. Bureau of the Census, 1980 Census, cited in *Boston Globe*, Feb. 25, 1982.

13. Emmett B. Keeler, David Solomon, John C. Beck, Robert Mendenhall, and Robert Kane, "Effect of Patient Age on Duration of Medical Encounters with Physicians," *Medical Care* XX, no. 11 (November 1982).

14 Cost Elements in Alternative Settings

Mary G. Henderson and
Fay L. Hannon

The disparity in third-party reimbursement for ambulatory health services between hospital OPDs and private physicians' offices is increasingly being questioned by policymakers. One study in Vermont found that hospitals were reimbursed an average of $26 under Medicaid for treating the common cold whereas private physicians' total payment averaged $8.75 for the same condition.[1] The crux of the problem is determining whether such differentials in reimbursement are justified on the basis of differentials in cost and, if so, what exactly are payers getting for their money in hospital settings. Solving this problem is critical: Hospitals have become heavily involved in the delivery of primary care, and this trend is likely to continue.[2]

The issue of why it is more costly to deliver ambulatory care in a hospital setting has generated much controversy. Few studies contain explicit comparisons of ambulatory-care costs across sites, and those that are available are limited in scope and are generally plagued with methodological defects and data-quality problems.[3] The explanations that have been advanced to account for the cost differential between hospital OPDs, particularly those in teaching hospitals, and physicians' private practices have centered on three major factors:

1. The hospital is producing a different product.
2. Cost measurement in the hospital overallocates overhead to the hospital OPD.
3. The hospital setting in and of itself generates higher outpatient costs due to the codeliverance of costly and complex inpatient care.

The first factor, or "product-difference" argument, encompasses the possibility that hospitals provide a more complex mix of services to outpatients, partially because the OPD sees a more complex mix of patients than private physicians and partially because the presence of highly trained personnel and technically sophisticated equipment leads to more expensive, resource-intensive, and (perhaps) higher quality care. Another aspect of this argument concerns teaching and research activities; teaching hospitals

This research has been supported by the Robert Wood Johnson Foundation, Grant 5180, and by the Health Care Financing Administration, Grant 18–P/97905.

can be said to be producing teaching and research services along with patient care. The attendant costs of such activities are included in the cost of an OPD patient visit, perhaps leading to higher per-visit costs.

Several studies investigating hospital cost-allocation systems have indicated that statistical changes in the way costs are apportioned to the inpatient and outpatient cost centers can significantly alter outpatient per-visit costs. Some writers have suggested that the use of allocation bases that more accurately reflect actual resource use would result in lower outpatient costs.[4,5,6] Another related phenomenon that could contribute to higher allocated costs in the OPD concerns how cost centers are defined. For example, third-party payer cost reports typically allow for only a small number of profit centers to which all overhead costs must be allocated. Intensity of use of these overhead services are usually not taken into account. Thus, ancillary services, a source of major revenue and an intensive user of some overhead services, for example, medical records, is typically not allocated its full share of overhead costs compared to outpatient services, which is overallocated.[7]

The third factor has been identified by Schultz as "by-product costs." These result from the OPDs being located in the same financial system with the more complex and extensive inpatient services. For example, a private physician's group practice may incur some minor expenses for security services; in contrast, the hospital is likely to have an entire security department, and the portion of its cost borne by the OPD may result in a more expensive way of providing the same type of security services. Also included here are stand-by costs that reflect the costs of the twenty-four hour availability of certain services.

In this chapter, we have attempted to compare the average cost per visit between the hospital OPD and private-physician group practice. The analysis does not attempt to provide an exhaustive nor completely controlled comparison of ambulatory-care costs across sites. For example, major components of the cost per visit, namely, the physician cost per visit and the ancillary cost per visit, have been excluded. Major aspects of the first factor listed earlier, that is, the product difference between the OPD and private physicians' offices, are beyond the scope of this analysis. These include potential differences in the medical and/or socioeconomic case mix of patients seen in the two sites and possible differences in the quality of care. (See Lion for a comparison of medical case mix[8] and Lion and Williams for a discussion of socioeconomic differences across sites of care.[9]) Finally, the two data sources that we have used in our comparison are drawn from different populations: the hospital OPD data is from the state of California while the group-practice data is from a national sample. But, as will be explained later, we have taken steps to compare our California hospitals with all U.S. hospitals and the national group-practice data with California group practices.

In spite of the aforementioned limitations of our analysis, we have undertaken it because of the important insights that have been obtained about the nonphysician cost differential between hospital OPDs and private-physician group practice. We have been able to partially address the product-difference argument through a detailed breakdown and comparison of the expense categories of the average visit to an OPD and to a private physician's office. Differences in the visit product can be inferred through a comparison of the type and wage rates of nonphysician personnel across sites of care. Our data also allow us to separate teaching costs per visit from other overhead costs in the hospital; the magnitude of this expense can also be estimated.

The data set from which hospital outpatient cost per visit was calculated is based on principles of uniform accounting. The statistical-allocation bases are highly accurate, and the cost groups are narrowly defined. The cost information provided on these reports is not used for reimbursement purposes. The use of these data circumvents much of the problems of cost measurement that other studies have encountered.

The cost-categorization methodology that we used permitted a determination of the amount of hospital-overhead cost that would not be present in a private physician's group practice. We have chosen to call these costs *noncounterpart* costs. The magnitude of these noncounterpart costs allows an estimation of by-product costs or those that occur because the OPD is located in a facility mainly designed to produce complicated, inpatient care.

Data Sources

The hospital OPD data consists of all hospitals reporting to the California Health Facilities Commission (CHFC) in FY 1979 that met the following criteria: (1) the type of care was short-term general, children's or university/teaching; (2) clinic costs were reported; and (3) more than 1,000 clinic visits were reported. Hospitals were also omitted that were found to have only one or two specialized, non-primary-care clinics (for example, dentistry).

The CHFC data base was chosen because it contains detailed cost information that is reported uniformly by law to a state agency. It is not used for reimbursement purposes. Although we realize that some bias and inaccuracies may be present in these data, they are considered superior to the Medicare cost reports, the only other large-scale body of cost data available. Table 14–1 shows a comparison of the hospitals with OPDs reporting to the CHFC with similar hospitals reporting to the American Hospital Association (AHA) for California and for the United States as a whole.

Information from the CHFC was selected for analysis because it was considered to be less biased than Medicare cost report information. We were surprised to learn, however, that the composition of California institu-

Table 14-1

Comparison of Hospital Outpatient Department Visits, California and United States

Hospital Characteristics	California Health Facilities Commission		California American Hospital Association		U.S. American Hospital Association	
	Number	Percent	Number	Percent	Number	Percent
Hospitals						
Nonteaching						
Under 400 beds	57	54%	187	75	1,754	67
400 beds or more	3	3	6	2	89	3
Teaching						
Under 400 beds	30	28	34	14	379	15
400 beds or more	16	15	23	9	384	15
Total	106	100	250	100	2,606	100
Visits						
Nonteaching						
Under 400 beds	869,209	14	4,306,997	44	30,619,772	33
400 beds or more	69,560	1	298,076	3	3,175,539	4
Teaching						
Under 400 beds	2,158,869	35	2,447,261	25	20,349,404	22
400 beds or more	3,070,535	50	2,801,709	38	37,726,036	41
Total	6,168,173	100	9,854,043	100	91,870,751	100

tions reporting CHFC information differs substantially from those that report to the AHA.

As shown in table 14-1 the AHA data indicates that 250 hospitals in California operate OPDs. In comparison, only 106 institutions are included in the CHFC analysis. Reasons for this difference include the fact that Kaiser-Permanente hospitals are not required to report financial data to CHFC, study staff excluded hospitals with fewer than 1,000 OPD visits, and, about 15 hospitals provided data that were inadequate for our analysis. Finally, the AHA classifies OPDs in short-term specialty hospitals and school health services as "short-term general" while study staff has eliminated these institutions from the CHFC analysis.

These differences explain, in part, the substantially higher proportion of teaching-hospital OPD visits as reported by CHFC (85 percent) compared to the 53 percent in the AHA survey of California institutions. But the major difference appears to be the *exclusion* by the AHA of the largest teaching hospital in the state from their universe, as well as 26 smaller hospitals.

The teaching hospital in question is Los Angeles County, University of Southern California Medical Center, which reported 1.5 million OPD visits and complete financial data on its OPD operations to CHFC but reported that it did not have an OPD at all to AHA. The difficulty appears to be with the spin-off to a separate corporation of the OPD by this hospital that enables it to answer the AHA question negatively but still requires it to report to CHFC.

Recalculating the AHA data to include LAC-USC Medical Center (which accounts for over 90 percent of the discrepancy in visits) raises the percent of OPD visits to large teaching hospitals in California to 38 percent compared with 50 percent for CHFC. Alternately, eliminating LAC-USC from the CHFC data base reduces the percent of OPD visits in large teaching hospitals from 50 to 33 percent compared with 28 percent for all California hospitals with OPDs.

In summary, the CHFC data tends to underrepresent somewhat the experience of small nonteaching hospitals compared to the nation as a whole. But the discrepancy is far less than to be expected by simply comparing CHFC data with the AHA California universe. Given the wide variation of per-visit costs for the small hospitals with OPDs that we did analyze, we feel reasonably confident that the sample used in this study is a more accurate reflection of the average cost of OPD visits in California. Further, the overall findings of the cost study are so strong that it is highly probable that they reflect the general tendencies for the country as a whole.

The private physician group practice data was obtained from an aggregation of information from the Medical Group Management Association (MGMA) 1981 Financial Management and Cost Survey. The MGMA had 171 group practices respond to both their surveys in 1981. Of these groups, which are located across the United States, 122 are free standing and reported usable data.

The MGMA comprises group practices containing three or more physicians, with an average of twenty-four physicians. Of the 122 free-standing groups, 72 percent are multispecialty, and most are located in mid-sized cities. The mean number of visits to an MGMA clinic is over 95,000.

Fourteen of the MGMA groups with usable data are located in California. These groups are slightly larger than average, with a mean number of 28 physicians and 106,000 clinic visits. A slightly smaller proportion, 58 percent, are multispecialty.

Cost Comparison

Table 14–2 presents the average nonphysician cost per visit for the CHFC hospital OPD data and for the MGMA group practice data. The average total nonphysician cost in the OPD is $36.92 versus $22.17 for the physician group practice, a 66-percent difference. The hospital costs have been split

Table 14–2

Comparison of Average Nonphysician Cost per Visit in Hospital Outpatient Departments to Large Group Practices

Cost Components	Hospital OPD	Physician's Group Practice
Direct Expenses		
Clinic salaries and benefits	$8.66	4.91
G&A salaries and benefits	8.20	5.56
Physician and student compensation[a]	.71	—
Contracted services	1.12	1.08
Supplies	1.69	2.53
Other	1.71	1.82
Adjustments	(−.36)	—
Total Direct	$21.73	$15.90
Allocated Expenses		
Counterpart[b]		
Clinical support	1.36	—
General and administrative	4.45	—
Plant	6.24	6.27
Total allocated counterpart	12.05	6.27
Total visit related	$33.78	$22.17
Noncounterpart[c]		
Special hospital services, clinical	1.20	
Special hospital services, G&A	1.18	
Inpatient support	.56	
Research and education	1.15	
Transfers	(−.95)	
Total allocated noncounterpart	$3.14	—
Average total cost	$36.92	$22.17

Note: Inflation adjusted to fiscal year ending June 30, 1980.

[a]This category contains the cost of non-patient-care activities performed by physicians, interns, and residents. The corresponding figure is not available from the group-practice data.

[b]Services that are also present in a physician's office.

[c]Services unique to a hospital-based setting.

into three major categories: direct, allocated counterpart, and allocated noncounterpart. Allocated-counterpart costs are those overhead costs that would also be incurred in a group-practice setting. Examples include plant and medical-records expenses. This category comprises 33 percent of total average cost. Allocated-noncounterpart costs are those that have no equivalent in the private setting. Research, education, and cafeteria expenses are examples of noncounterpart-allocated costs. Over 8 percent of total average cost can be attributed to these noncounterpart costs. Appendixes 14A and 14B contain a detailed classification of hospital expenses.

The expenses reported by the group practices were considered to pertain to one cost center, and so the total is actually $22.17 in direct cost. For comparability, however, the $6.27 plant cost is shown in the allocated category.

Table 14-3 presents a comparison of the hospital OPD and group practice costs in which the clinical-support and general-and-administrative costs (counterpart categories) have been distributed to the direct-expense categories based on the proportion of direct clinic cost in each category. This distribution of counterpart costs is undertaken to achieve the greatest comparability between the OPD and private practice sites' cost components.

As table 14-3 shows, the hospital OPD average cost is $14.66 higher than the group-practice average cost. Of this difference, 78 percent is due to the OPD having higher salary costs. (Note that even before the clinical-support and general-administrative cost categories from table 14-2 were distributed to the direct-expense categories, salary costs in the OPD are still 61 percent higher than the group-practice costs.) Surprisingly, the only other significant cost component, plant cost, is virtually identical between the two sites. The remaining 21 percent of the difference is attributed to the non-counterpart costs.

The major differential observed in salary costs across sites appears to result from more personnel, higher salaries, and a different mix of personnel in the OPD as compared to the group-practice setting. A more detailed breakdown of salary expenses by personnel type will be presented later in this paper. First, an examination of how the cost components vary by size of the delivery site will be undertaken.

Table 14-3
Comparison of Hospital Outpatient Department and
Large-Group-Practice Cost per Visit,[a] by Cost Components

Cost Components	Hospital OPDs (Dollars)	Physician's Group Practice (Dollars)	Difference (Dollars)	Percent OPDs Are Higher
Clinic support salaries and benefits	9.99	4.91	5.08	103
General and administrative salaries	12.04	5.56	6.48	117
Contracted services	1.44	1.08	0.36	33
Supplies	2.23	2.53	(0.30)	(−12)
Other	1.84	1.82	0.02	1
Plant	6.24	6.27	(0.03)	—
Total	33.78	22.17	11.52	52
Noncounterpart	3.14	—	—	—
Grand total	36.92	22.17	14.66	66

[a]Inflation adjusted to fiscal year ending June 30, 1980.

The Influence of Size on Cost per Visit

Tables 14–4 and 14–5 present the average nonphysician cost per visit calculated for three categories of size of the delivery site. Hospital size is measured by number of beds, and in table 14–5, group practice size by the number of full-time equivalent physicians.

Turning first to the hospitals, it is of considerable interest that the largest hospitals' nonphysician cost per visit of $49.41 is twice as high as the $24.81 average total cost for the small hospitals and 41 percent higher than the $35.14 for the mid-sized hospitals. Interestingly, the proportion of total nonphysician cost per visit that is classified as direct cost increases from 53 percent in the small hospitals to 60 percent in the mid-sized hospitals and 62 percent in the large. Similarly, direct cost increases 133 percent from the small to large bed-size category while total allocated average cost only shows a 61-percent jump. This finding seems to contradict the common assumption that it is overhead costs in larger hospitals that account for the greater cost per visit. However, it is not possible to determine the extent to which this

Table 14–4
Average Nonphysician Cost per Hospital Outpatient Department Visit Categorized by Hospital Bed Size

Cost Components	Small	Medium	Large
Direct Expenses			
Clinic salaries and benefits	$ 6.13	$ 8.47	$11.26
G&A salaries and benefits	3.88	8.30	12.05
Other direct	3.20	4.26	7.48
Total direct	13.21	21.03	30.79
Allocated Expenses			
Counterpart[a]			
Plant	4.14	6.39	7.62
Other counterpart	4.97	5.77	6.21
Total counterpart	9.11	12.16	13.83
Noncounterpart[b]			
Research and education	0.67	1.22	1.54
Other noncounterpart	1.82	0.73	3.25
Total noncounterpart	2.49	1.95	4.79
Total allocated	11.60	14.11	18.62
Average total cost	$24.81	$35.14	$49.41

Note: Inflation adjusted to fiscal year ending June 30, 1980. *Small* consists of thirty-four hospitals under 130 beds; *medium*, thirty-seven hospitals from 130 to 299 beds; and *large*, thirty-four hospitals of 300 beds or more.
[a]Services that are also present in a physician's office.
[b]Services unique to a hospital-based setting.

Table 14–5
Comparison of Personnel Costs per Patient Visit, Type of Personnel and Hospital Bed Size

Salary Costs (Excluding Benefits)	Size of Hospital			Total
	Small	Medium	Large	
Cost per Visit				
Patient-care practitioners[a]	$3.32	$ 3.71	$ 3.97	$ 3.67
Management, supervision, and clerical	2.78	5.21	6.19	4.73
Technical and specialists	1.13	2.56	4.01	2.57
Other	0.06	0.10	0.46	0.21
Total	$7.29	$11.58	$14.63	$11.18
Hourly Rate				
Patient-care practitioners[a]	$6.51	$ 7.07	$ 7.41	$ 7.03
Management, supervision, and clerical	6.79	7.68	7.53	7.43
Technical specialists	8.27	8.43	8.11	8.25
Other	7.26	6.26	5.79	6.15
Hours per Visit				
Patient-care practitioners[a]	0.49	0.52	0.54	0.65
Management, supervision, and clerical	0.50	0.76	0.89	0.72
Technical and specialists	0.18	0.25	0.50	0.31
Other	0.01	0.01	0.09	0.04

[a]Includes RNs, LVNs, aides, orderlies, and other nonphysician practitioners.

finding is due to the common practice of large hospitals to charge more expenses directly to departments.

Direct Expenses

For hospitals of all three sizes, most of the direct expenses come from salaries. The proportion of direct expenses that are salaries remains fairly constant at between 76 and 80 percent. Clinical-support salaries and benefits almost double from the small to large bed-size categories, while general-and-administrative salaries and benefits more than triple. It is clear that personnel costs account for most of the difference in the nonphysician cost of providing an OPD visit across bed-size categories.

The CHFC data base is unique in that it presents detailed information about hours and wage rates of many different classifications of personnel. A disaggregation of the total cost of four personnel categories into hourly rates and productive hours per visit is presented in table 14–5. The total non-physician-personnel cost per visit is twice as high in the large versus the small hospitals. Most of the difference is due to the higher administrative per-visit cost and technical and specialist per-visit cost.

Interestingly, the patient-care practitioner cost remains fairly constant across hospital bed-size categories. The average hourly rate for patient-care practitioners increases less than $1.00 from the small to large hospital size category, and the average (mean) productive hours per visit does not increase significantly. In contrast, the productive hours per visit for administrative personnel and for the technical specialists shows a large jump from the small to large bed-size category while the wage rate remains fairly constant. It is thus the time spent per visit, not the hourly rate, that accounts for the higher personnel costs in the larger hospitals.

Overhead Expenses

Referring back to table 14–4, we note that in contrast to the direct expenses, total allocated costs fall from 47 percent to 38 percent of total nonphysician per-visit cost from the small to large hospitals. Thus, contrary to the conventional wisdom, OPDs located in larger, presumably more complicated hospitals do not appear to be bearing a larger portion of overhead than OPDs in smaller hospitals. (As previously mentioned, however, it is unclear the extent to which different accounting practices explain this difference). The allocated expenses that are "counterpart," that is, do have an equivalent in a physician's office, account for over three-quarters of total allocated expenses in all three size categories. Plant costs account for 45 percent of these allocated, counterpart expenses in the small hospitals, 53 percent in the mid-sized, and 55 percent in the large. Thus, as would be expected, OPDs in larger hospitals due to their location in larger cities and in more complicated physical plants, have a slightly higher proportion of per-visit plant expenses.

Noncounterpart Costs

Noncounterpart costs, or expenses that do not occur in a free-standing ambulatory-care setting, show an interesting pattern. As shown in table 14–4, these costs account for approximately 10 percent of total nonphysician cost per visit in the small and large hospitals and roughly 6 percent of per visit cost in the mid-sized hospitals. While the magnitude of these costs is not overwhelming, it is important to realize that most OPD visits occur in larger hospitals. In California almost $5.00 of the per-visit nonphysician cost in the largest hospitals represents an expense for services that would not be supplied at all in a private physician's office. These noncounterpart expenses are incurred because the OPD is part of a larger institution providing costly inpatient services; thus their magnitude represents an estimation of by-product costs.

Research and Education

A special subcategory of noncounterpart costs, those due to research and education, is worthy of special attention because of its important health-policy implications. These expenses constitute 3 percent of total nonphysician average cost across all three size categories (see table 14–2).

Teaching hospitals have consistently been reported as having higher OPD costs than nonteaching hospitals. Based on a typology of teaching hospitals developed for a study commissioned by the Department of Health and Human Services, CHFC hospitals were divided into categories based on graduate medical involvement. As shown in table 14–6, the average total cost increases from a cost of $34.93 at the low commitment level to $45.21 at the high level of teaching involvement.

Direct costs increase by 18 percent from the low to high teaching

Table 14–6
Mean Nonphysician Total Cost, by Level of Commitment to Graduate Medical Education

Cost Components	Commitment to GME		Total
	Low	High	
Average Nonphysician Cost			
Direct	$21.13	$25.01	$21.73
Research and Education	0.95	2.16	1.15
Other allocated	12.85	18.04	14.04
Total	34.93	45.21	36.92
Average Bed Size	209	497	255
Number of Hospitals	89	17	106

Note: Inflation adjusted to fiscal year ending June 30, 1980. Data based on a typology from "A Study of the Financing of Graduate Medical Education: Development of a Typology of Teaching Hospitals" (Policy Analysis, Inc., 1981, unpublished). In order to construct this typology, data were collected on several variables considered relevant to assessing the degree of commitment to graduate medical education (number of residents in different specialty training programs, number of teaching faculty) from hospitals reporting any type of medical-teaching activity to the American Hospital Association. These data were subjected to a cluster analysis that yielded five different levels of teaching involvement. The two highest levels and the three lowest levels have been combined in this analysis. Hospitals with a low level of commitment are those with zero or one residency program, while those at the high end of the spectrum have many. Note that the research-and-education cost category from the CHFC data set includes the costs of nursing and paramedical-education activities.

commitment while allocated costs show a 40-percent increase. As one would expect, costs specifically designated as pertaining to research-and-education activities more than double, from under \$1.00 in hospitals with little or no commitment to teaching and research to over \$2.00 in advanced teaching hospitals. Considering that most OPD visits in California and in the United States as a whole occur in teaching hospitals (see table 14–1), \$2.00 per visit means that a significant portion of private and public payment for out-patient care is channeled into research-and-education activities.

Group Practice Costs

Table 14–7 presents a breakdown of the average nonphysician cost by group-practice size, measured by full-time equivalent physicians. Although the large group practices have higher average costs than the smaller ones, the difference is not as striking as the hospital-size difference. Large group practices have average costs 25 percent greater than small groups and 31 percent higher than mid-sized groups. Interestingly, the mid-sized groups appear to be the least expensive. Most of the average cost difference—42 percent—between the mid-sized and large groups is due to lower plant costs in the mid-sized groups. This again is in contrast to the hospitals, where 54 percent of the cost difference due to size arose from higher salary costs in the larger hospitals.

It is interesting to compare the group-practice costs with those of the small OPDs. It is reasonable to believe that the product produced in these two sites may be similar. However, the average nonphysician cost per visit in

Table 14–7
Average Nonphysician Cost per Private-Physician Group-Practice Visit Categorized by Group-Practice Size in Physician Full-time Equivalents

Cost Components	Small	Medium	Large	Total
Clinic support salaries and benefits	\$ 3.65	\$ 4.03	\$ 4.92	\$ 4.22
General and administrative salaries	5.39	5.13	6.14	5.56
Contracted services	1.16	1.01	1.07	1.08
Supplies	2.43	2.13	3.02	2.53
Other	1.75	1.54	2.15	1.82
Plant	5.67	5.29	7.78	6.27
Total	\$20.05	\$19.13	\$25.08	\$21.48

Note: Inflation adjusted to fiscal year ending June 30, 1980. *Small* equals 10 or less FTE physicians; *medium* equals more than 10 and less than 22.5 FTE physicians; *large* equals greater than 22.5 FTE physicians.

the group-practice data of $21.48 is lower than even the small hospital cost of $24.81 (from table 14–4). It is also apparent that the individual components of cost show differences between the group practices and the small hospitals. For example, salary costs (distributed) in the small hospitals are approximately $14.00 compared to $9.78 in the group practices. Plant costs in the small OPDs are $4.14 versus $6.27 for the group practices. Thus the pattern of costs between the two sites seems to suggest that the product produced in the two sites is different. However, without detailed information about patient case mix and specific clinic services provided, this is only speculation.

Conclusion

This comparison between hospital OPD and physician group-practice non-physician costs has uncovered several points of interest about the cost of ambulatory-care delivery in alternative sites. Insights into the issue are becoming increasingly important as the federal government continues to propose funding mechanisms for ambulatory services that reimburse hospitals at the same rate as free-standing facilities.

Not surprisingly, the average nonphysician-cost per visit in the hospital was found to be significantly higher than the group-practice, per-visit cost. Furthermore, most of the cost difference (79 percent) between sites of care was due to higher salary costs in the hospital OPD. The per-visit costs for supplies and for plant were strikingly similar. The remaining cost differential was generated by the presence of the noncounterpart costs in the hospital OPD. Thus a small but significant proportion of the average nonphysician cost difference was caused by the presence of services and activities in the hospital that are not found in private group practice. Particularly in large hospitals, where the great majority of OPD visits occur, noncounterpart costs account for almost $5.00 per visit. Research and education costs, a special category of noncounterpart costs, were found to be a significant cost component for advanced teaching hospitals, averaging over $2.00 per visit.

This seemingly small amount for research and education becomes significant in considering the fact that teaching hospitals have recently engaged in a large expansion of their primary-care clinics in order to provide residencies in family-practice and other related specialties.

While our data is not detailed enough to allow us to consider case-mix differences and clinic-services differences across our two data sets, it is likely that these differences do occur. The question then becomes one of estimating this differential and determining whether the observed cost differences can be justified by them (see chapter 13).

When we examined the cost data broken down by the size of the delivery site, the hospital OPDs showed clear and striking average-cost differences across bed-size categories while the group-practice data did not. Again, most of the cost differential between the small and large hospitals was due to administrative and technical specialists' salary costs. Interestingly, the hours per visit, not the wage rate, appeared to account for most of the difference. Clearly, the larger hospitals are either expending more personnel resources per visit or have more personnel on hand. Without more detailed studies, it is not possible to know which situation is actually occurring. Unfortunately, the group-practice data did not allow a disaggregation of total salary costs into wage rates and hours. Because most of the cost difference between the two sites was due to salaries, the lack of this information for the group-practice data is an important missing piece of the puzzle. Further research should be undertaken in this area.

Notes

1. Gail Rotegard, et al., *A Service Delivery Assessment of Medicaid Payments for Hospital Out-patient Services in Vermont* (Boston: Office of Service Delivery Assessment, U.S. Department of Health, Education and Welfare Region I, November 1979).

2. Timothy A. Stalker, "What's Behind the Explosive Growth in Hospital-Based Primary Care?" *Hospital Physician*, Part I, February 1979; Part II, March 1979.

3. Marsha Gold, "Hospital-based versus Free-standing Primary Care Costs," *Journal of Ambulatory Care Medicine* 2, no. 1 (February 1979).

4. Arne Anderson and Daniel Zwick, "Improving the Methods Used to Determine Hospital Ambulatory Service Costs," National Center for Health Services Research (Paper delivered at the Annual Meeting of the American Public Health Association, Washington, D.C., Statistics Section, 1977).

5. B. Schultz, "An Analysis of Hospital Care Ambulatory Costs," (Ph.D. dis., New York University, 1975).

6. David W. Young, et al., "Ambulatory Care Costs and the Medicare Cost Report: Managerial and Public Policy Implications," *Journal of Ambulatory Care Management* 5, no. 1 (February 1982):

7. Judy Smith, et al., "Determining the True Cost of Hospital-Based Ambulatory Care," *Journal of Ambulatory Care Management* 6, no. 1 (February 1983):

8. Joanna Lion, "Commentaries: Case Mix Differences Among Ambulatory Patients Seen by Internists in Various Settings," *Health Services Research* 16, no. 4 (winter 1981):

9. See chapter 13 in this volume.

Appendix 14A
Cost-Categorization
Scheme

Clinic Costs (per Clinic Line of Trial Balance)

1. Clinical salaries and benefits
2. G&A salaries and benefits
3. Physician and student compensation (excluding compensation for patient care)
4. Contracted services
5. Supplies
6. Other
7. Adjustments

Costs Allocated to the Clinic (per Stepdown)

Counterpart

8. Clinical support
9. G&A
10. Plant

Noncounterpart

11. Special hospital services, clinical
12. Special hospital services, G&A
13. Inpatient support
14. Research and education
15. Transfers

Note: This classification scheme is taken from the California Health Facilities Commission hospital cost report.

Appendix 14B
Classification of
Allocated Expenses

Counterpart Costs

8. Clinical Support
   8350 Laundry and linen
   8690 Medical library
   8700 Medical records
   7050 Central services
   7170 Pharmacy

9. General and Administrative
   8860 Working-capital interest
   8610 Hospital administration
   8510 General accounting
   8520 Communications
   8310 Printing and duplication
   8650 Personnel
   8420 Purchasing and stores
   8530 Patient accounting
   8540 Data processing
   8550 Credit and collection
   8830 Professional liability insurance

10. Plant
   8870 Interest
   8840 Insurance, except professional liability
   8850 Licenses and taxes
   8810 Depreciation and amortization
   8820 Leases and rentals
   8460 Housekeeping
   8430 Grounds
   8470 Plant operations
   8480 Plant maintenance
   8490 Other general operations

Noncounterpart Costs

11. Special Hospital Services, Clinical
   8710 Medical staff
   8360 Social services

8720 Nursing administration
8740 Inservice education, nursing

12. Special Hospital Services, G&A
    8620 Governing board
    8630 Public relations
    8640 Management engineering
    8750 Other administrative services
    8570 Other fiscal services
    8660 Employee medical-services administration
    8880 Employee benefits, nonpayroll
    8330 Cafeteria
    8440 Security
    8450 Parking
    8890 Other unassigned costs
    8400 Other retail operations

13. Inpatient Support
    8380 Employee housing
    8340 Dietary
    8670 Auxiliary groups
    8680 Chaplaincy services
    8560 Admitting
    8390 Physicians' offices and other rentals

14. Research and Education
    8010 Research administrative office
    8020 Research projects
    8030 Other research
    8210 Education administration office
    8260 Student housing
    8230 LVN program
    8220 School of nursing
    8250 Paramedical education
    8270 Other education activities
    8240 Medical postgraduate education

15

Medicaid Costs, Ambulatory-Care Setting, and Hospital Use

Philip J. Held and
Katherine Swartz

Total national expenditures for the Medicaid program increased 237 percent between 1973 and 1979—or an average annual compound rate of growth of 14.4 percent.[1] Even after allowance is made for the growth in the number of Medicaid recipients (10 percent between 1973 and 1979) and inflation in medical-care prices (74 percent between 1973 and 1979),[2] program costs still grew at an average annual compound rate of growth of 7.3 percent. Increases of this magnitude generated considerable policy interest and helped instigate the rather dramatic changes in the Medicaid program after President Reagan took office in 1980.

The growth in Medicaid expenditures for the 1973–79 period varied by type of service, with hospital outpatient services growing at the largest rate of 19 percent per year, doubling in less than four years.[3] However, hospital outpatient services were only 4 percent of the total program costs in 1979, and just under 16 percent of all ambulatory costs. By contrast, short-term hospital expenditures accounted for 28 percent of total Medicaid expenditures in 1979. Not only are short-term hospital expenditures the largest single category of costs but their increases (13 percent per year compounded) have been dramatically rapid too.

Hospital use is of fundamental policy interest not only because of hospital expenditures' share of the budget but also because many have argued that hospital use is one of the most amendable sections of the health-care industry. Of particular interest is the relationship between the different settings for ambulatory care and short-term hospitalization expenses. Our study focuses on this relationship by examining the expenditures and health-care-use patterns for two groups of Medicaid eligibles in California between 1976 and 1978.[4]

In brief, our findings are that as a proportion of total expenditures per

This research was supported by Grant 18–P–97516/3–01, Health Care Financing Administration, U.S. Department of Health and Human Services. Opinions expressed are those of the authors and do not necessarily represent the views of The Urban Institute or its sponsors. The excellent research assistance of Carol Hamcke is gratefully acknowledged. Robert Berenson, M.D., and Helen Smits, M.D., were both very resourceful and helpful in the classification of diagnoses and procedures.

eligible, in-patient care in short-term hospitals accounts for by far the largest share, with almost half of all expenditures. By contrast, ambulatory physician care accounted for about 8 percent of total expenditures per eligible for the disabled and 17 percent for the AFDC females. When we examine hospitalization rates across the different ambulatory-care settings, there are striking differences. For example, an AFDC female whose predominant source of ambulatory care (PSC) is an outpatient department (OPD) of a hospital is nearly twice as likely to be hospitalized as her counterpart whose PSC is a private physician's office. This appears to contradict the findings of Lion and Altman who have argued that there are no substantial case-mix differences between patients seen in private practice and OPDs, at least for patients seen by primary-care practitioners. But our different hospitalization rates lead to an obvious question: Are certain ambulatory-care settings simply more willing to hospitalize patients, or can at least some of these differences be accounted for by differences in the health status of patients who use these different settings?

The plan of this chapter is first to describe the data used for this study and then to give the distributions of predominant source of care (PSC) for the two study samples. Next expenditures and hospitalization rates will be compared according to PSC. Hospital-discharge diagnoses are then investigated to help clarify why the hospitalization rates are so different by PSC. Finally, the importance of these descriptive findings, particularly in terms of how they relate to reimbursement policy will be discussed.[5]

Data

The data presented here were computed from eligibility and medical-claims records for two groups of the California Medicaid (Medi-Cal) population. The first group consisted of nonaged (under sixty-five years of age), female, AFDC–cash-assistance recipients excluding the seven- to fourteen-year-old cohort and all recipients living in Los Angeles County. The sample for this group was drawn from Medi-Cal eligibility records in a manner that oversampled for two age cohorts (less than one year, and fifty to sixty-four year olds) and rural counties. The data presented have been corrected, however, for age and geographic stratification. While the total sample drawn was approximately 50,000 per year for the AFDC sample and 10,000 per year for the disabled, the data presented here were based on smaller subsamples.

The second group consisted of the disabled, again excluding those who lived in Los Angeles County. The sample for this group was a systematic random sample of the Medi-Cal eligibles. The data presented in this chapter are based on 8,622 female AFDC and 8,151 disabled eligibles evenly distributed over the three years 1976–1978.

Predominant Source of Care

Predominant source of care (PSC) is intended to reflect the type of setting in which an individual receives ambulatory medical care (physician visits). Our presumption is that the PSC reflects a beneficiary's usual point of entry into the health-care system.

A PSC was assigned to each Medicaid eligible who had an ambulatory physician visit on the basis of the frequency of visits that the person had to each of the various settings over a six-month period; the setting with the highest number of visits by the individual was selected as the PSC for that person. Two levels of aggregation of the PSC were used. The first used four settings: private physician's office; OPD in a hospital; an emergency room (ER) in a hospital; and a clinic, which is generally a multiservice, free-standing entity. The second level of aggregation divided the private physician's office into general practice and specialist, and the hospital OPDs and ERs into public- and private. Each of the levels of aggregation also accounted for the nonusers, that is, people who received no ambulatory physician visits during the six months. Including nonusers as a separate category ensures that all eligibles are included in one of the mutually exclusive categories. A person could, of course, use medical care such as inpatient hospital care without being a user of ambulatory physician visits, although such occurrences are rare. In general, this chapter focuses on the greater level of aggregation, that is, the four settings of care, since the level of precision with the eight settings of care is frequently inadequate for our purposes.

Tables 15–1 and 15–2 show the overall distributions of PSC as well as the distributions of PSC by age, sex, and rural residence in 1976 and 1978, for the female AFDC eligibles and the disabled eligibles, respectively. An overview of tables 15–1 and 15–2 shows substantial similarities in the patterns of where these two groups receive their ambulatory care. For both groups, more than half received ambulatory care in private physicians' offices, a proportion that is roughly comparable to the national average.[6] This was also the case for those who lived in the rural areas. The proportion who used OPDs and ERs was also similar for both the disabled and the AFDC females.

Perhaps the most striking difference between these two groups of eligibles appears in the age distributions; this is not surprising, however, given the different eligibility requirements for the two groups. Almost half the disabled are between fifty and sixty-four years old, whereas only 3 percent of the AFDC females are in this age cohort. Similarly, only slightly more than 1 percent of the disabled are less than six years old, but just over a fourth of the AFDC females are less than six years old. Another striking difference between the two groups is the proportion who are nonusers of ambulatory

Table 15-1
Distribution of Predominant Source of Care, by Age, Year, and Geographic Location for Female AFDC Medicaid Eligibles, California, 1976-1978

Location	Year	Weight[b]	*Percent with Predominant Source of Care*[a]					
			Private Office	*ER*	*OPD*	*Clinic*	*Nonuser of Ambulatory Care*	*Total*
All	1976	100.0	58.0	9.4	6.9	2.5	23.5	100.0
	1978	100.0	57.4	8.2	8.3	3.6	22.5	100.0
"Rural" counties[c]	1976	11.9	55.4	8.3	6.2	4.0	26.1	100.0
	1978	12.3	50.2	7.3	7.6	9.1	25.8	100.0

Note: Data based on a sample of 8,622 female AFDC eligibles not eligible for prepaid care and eligible for at least six continuous months. Six age cohorts are included. Those seven to fourteen years old and those sixty-five or older are excluded. Los Angeles County and drug claims are excluded. Data are weighted to correct for age cohort and geographic stratification. Eligibles who received care in a long-term setting are not included in these data.

[a]Predominant source of care is defined as the setting where the maximum number of ambulatory physician visits occurred. ER is emergency room; OPD is outpatient department.
[b]Weight is the percent of the total sample, by year, in that row.
[c]"Rural" includes thirty-three counties with low population densities and few population centers.

Table 15-2
Distribution of Predominant Source of Care, by Age, Year, and Geographic Location for Disabled Medicaid Eligibles, California, 1976-1978

Location	Year	Weight[b]	*Percent with Predominant Source of Care*[a]					
			Private Office	*ER*	*OPD*	*Clinic*	*Nonuser of Ambulatory Care*	*Total*
All	1976	100.0	50.2	5.3	9.8	1.8	32.9	100.0
	1978	100.0	54.5	4.4	8.6	1.9	30.8	100.0
"Rural" counties[c]	1976	13.8	54.9	4.2	7.1	3.7	30.0	100.0
	1978	13.3	58.5	5.3	6.9	2.0	27.3	100.0
Female distribution	1976	53.2	57.1	4.3	10.5	2.0	26.2	100.0
Male distribution	1978	46.0	43.1	6.6	9.3	1.7	39.4	100.0

Note: Data based on a sample of 8,151 disabled eligibles. Those aged sixty-five years or older are excluded. Los Angeles County and drug claims are excluded. Eligibles who received care in a long-term setting are included in these data; 0.8 percent were missing data on their sex.

[a]Predominant source of care is defined as the setting where the maximum number of ambulatory physician visits occurred. ER is emergency room; OPD is outpatient department.
[b]The percent of the total sample, by year, in that row.
[c]"Rural" includes thirty-three counties with low population densities and few population centers.

physician visits: 23 percent of the AFDC females compared with 33 percent of the disabled in 1976.

Between 1976 and 1978 there were slight changes in the distribution of the PSC, and these changes differed across the two groups. While the AFDC females increased their use of the OPD and clinic, the disabled appeared to use the private physician's office more frequently. In addition, it appears that there was some decrease in the proportion of nonusers for the disabled, with essentially no change for the AFDC females. While these changes indicate trends that may or may not have continued over a longer period, essentially the basic overall pattern was unchanged over the three years. More refined analyses of the factors that affect the choice of a PSC setting will be found in Held and Swartz.[7]

Medicaid Costs and the Different Settings of Care

The overall pattern of expenditures (cost) for medical care and hospitalization for those eligibles whose PSC was either the private physician's office or the hospital OPD is shown in table 15–3. For both the disabled and the AFDC females, inpatient costs accounted for nearly half of the total cost per eligible of $251 and $521 for private office and OPD, respectively. (This total cost includes all care except drugs.) For both these groups, the hospitalization rate for patients whose PSC was an OPD was higher than the rate for patients whose PSC was a private physician's office. The differences across PSC in hospitalization rates were greater for the AFDC sample, in which beneficiaries whose predominant source of care was an OPD had a hospital-

Table 15–3
Mean Medicaid Cost per Eligible and Percent Hospitalized, by Eligibility and Source of Care, California, January–June, 1976–1978

Eligibility Status	Cost Parameter	Predominant Source of Care[a]		Total[b]
		Private Physician's Office	Hospital OPD	
Female AFDC	Percent hospitalized[c]	11	20	9
	Inpatient costs[d]	$130	$ 297	$121
	Percent of total	(44)	(62)	(48)
	Total costs	$296	$ 477	$251
Disabled	Percent hospitalized[c]	16	20	13
	Total inpatient costs	$296	$ 678	$318
	Percent of total	(53)	(68)	(61)
	Short term	$274	$ 501	$246
	Long term	$ 22	$ 177	$ 72
	Total costs	$555	$1,000	$521

Note: Data includes deliveries.
[a]Defined to be the setting where patients received most of their ambulatory physician visits.
[b]Includes all eligibles, not just the two sources of care shown here.
[c]Includes short- and long-term-care facilities. The latter are seldom used by AFDC females.
[d]Short-term facilities only.

ization rate that was almost twice that of beneficiaries whose PSC was a private physician's office. The differences in hospitalization rates across PSC for the disabled were also in the same direction but were not as large quantitatively (0.20 versus 0.16 hospitalized, or a difference of 25 percent). But the increased hospitalization naturally causes greater costs per beneficiary. In fact, for the AFDC sample, 92 percent of the difference of $181 in mean total cost between a private physician's office and an OPD is accounted for by the difference in the hospitalization rate. (Since the average length of stay and cost per hospital day are quite similar for patients from these two ambulatory settings, the difference is primarily determined by the proportion hospitalized.) For the disabled, the pattern is similar with differences in hospitalization costs accounting for 86 percent of the difference in mean total costs. Another significant part of the difference in cost for the disabled between private-office and OPD settings is the use of inpatient care other than short-term hospital, for example, long-term care.

These results are striking. In particular, they contradict stories claiming that OPDs are inherently more costly to Medicaid than other settings because of costs peculiar to the OPD (for example, social workers and hospital overhead). True, if one closely examines the data presented in this chapter, a case can be made that some services such as laboratory cost more per beneficiary in some settings than others. But in toto, these differences do not amount to a lot. The policy issue is clearly differences in hospitalization rates across different settings.

Given these proportionally large differences between the private physician's office and the hospital OPD in the total cost per beneficiary and the rate of hospitalizations, an obvious question arises: Why are beneficiaries from some PSC settings more likely to be hospitalized than beneficiaries from others?

Five potential explanations for these differences in hospitalization rates are shown in table 15–4. The first two focus on potential differences between either the patient or the physician. The third potential explanation has more to do with the general perception of OPDs as an institution for episodic care lacking in what might be called continuity or knowledge between the physician and the patient. The fourth explanation is more venal than the others. This explanation proposes that the hospital uses the OPD as a source of inpatients to fill hospital beds, that is, hospitalization occurs for economic reasons beyond what proper medical judgment would prescribe. A fifth explanation centers on pregnant women being more apt to use the OPD than a private practitioner for prenatal care.

It is frequently true that OPDs and other hospital settings such as the emergency room are staffed by medical residents, a fact that would provide some support to the first explanation. But is it true that residents are more likely to hospitalize patients than are other physicians? We do not know for

Table 15–4
Potential Explanations for Higher Hospitalization Rates for Outpatient Departments

Potential Explanation	Remarks
1. *Physicians* practicing in the OPDs are *different* from their counterparts in private offices in ways that lead to more conservative treatment.	1. E.g., younger or less-experienced physicians in OPDs.
2. *Patients* seen in hospital OPDs have a *different* health status than patients seen in private offices.	2. E.g., sicker or different presenting symptoms for OPD patients. Perhaps the OPD is a referral center.
3. Patients and physicians in the two settings may not be different, but the *interaction* in an OPD with its *episodic* care lacking continuity of patient-physician contact may lead to more conservative treatment in the OPD.	3. E.g., a physician does not know the parent of a sick child well enough to trust that the parent would contact the physician if conditions worsen. Consequently, the physician takes a more conservative approach and hospitalizes the child.
4. The OPD may be a source of inpatients, i.e., the OPD is the "side door" to the hospital, and the OPD is used to admit patients at a rate greater than required by proper medical practice.	
5. AFDC recipients seen in the OPD may be more likely to be pregnant and therefore to be hospitalized for delivery.	

sure, but anecdotal evidence would support this notion. The medical-claims data used in this project identified a physician's specialty but did not identify whether or not the physician was a medical resident in training. Consequently, we could not test this hypothesis.

Whether or not OPDs have a different case mix of patients compared to private practices is a major issue and has been addressed by Lion and Altman, among others.[8] Our approach is similar to some of the previous work but is different in significant ways; namely, we include visits to all specialties (Lion and Altman excluded visits to obstetricians and gynecologists), and we focus on both hospitalizations and procedures. Lion and Altman focused on the diagnosis for the ambulatory visit and the physician's assessment of severity. We will return to a comparison of our work with Lion and Altman in the next section.

The claims data we analyzed would not permit a step-by-step testing of each of the potential explanations. Consequently, we took a different approach and retrospectively categorized selected physician procedures for all beneficiaries and the hospital diagnoses of each of the Medicaid beneficiaries who were hospitalized. As we discuss this methodology in the next section, it will be seen that the results of this approach have some bearing on the potential hypotheses listed in table 15–4.

Discretion in the Choice of Hospitalization

A central focus of this study is the relationship between the setting in which a person receives ambulatory care and hospitalization—specifically, differences in hospitalization across different sources of care. The range of conditions for which patients are hospitalized is substantial, and there are cases when considerable discretion and judgment is required and conferred on the physician. For example, an acute appendicitis or the delivery of a baby does not permit much latitude for physician discretion about whether or not to hospitalize the patient. On the other hand, a hernia is normally subject to considerable discretion about whether to hospitalize and when. Because of these differences in the conditions presented for hospitalization, we have placed the hospital-discharge diagnoses into five a priori categories on the basis of the degree of discretion involved:

A. No discretion as to the need or when to hospitalize according to generally prevailing medical practice. This condition is generally not correlated with overall health status, for example, acute appendicitis or normal delivery.

B. Same as category A in that there is no discretion as to the need or timing of hospitalization, but the diagnoses are generally correlated with overall health status, for example, acute myocardial infarction or cerebral hemorrhage.

C. The decision to treat a condition that would require hospitalization is basically a quality-of-life choice. For example, surgery is discretionary to the extent that the condition is not life threatening but life would be more "comfortable" with the condition corrected. Normally, physicians would advise surgery for this condition provided a patient had medical insurance or the economic resources to pay for the medical care. The timing of the hospitalization is generally not urgent, for example, hernia, cataract or uterovaginal prolapse.

D. There is not enough information on the medical claim to classify the diagnosis. There is normally a range of severity of the medical diagnosis; and without more complete information on the individual patient and medical diagnosis than that presented on a medical claim, a retrospective classification of the diagnosis is not possible, for example, other bacterial diseases or other diseases of thyroid gland.

E. Treatment modality and hospitalization are open to choice and judgment depending on the diagnosis and individual patient severity, but it is not just a matter of information about the patient. These diagnoses represent medical conditions over which accepted medical opinion would permit choice of treatment modality or choice of treatment and would depend on patient severity even within given diagnoses, for example, diabetes mellitus, drug dependence or acute bronchitis.

F.   Discretion of the physician is required; however, the patient is usually not hospitalized for this condition, for example, mumps, chickenpox or acute tonsillitis.

Categories A and B are similar, although B may provide some measure of general-health status. While conceptually appealing, the frequencies of B diagnoses were so small that it was not likely to be a reliable measure. Consequently, we generally treat A and B as one category.

Categories C and E are similar in that both involve discretion and choice. But there is a distinct difference between them. Category C diagnoses generally do not permit choice about how to treat a given condition, only whether to treat, although a small fraction of the cases might permit choice about treatment setting. Category E, by contrast, contains conditions that permit both a decision of whether to treat and how to treat.

Categories D and E are similar in that in both cases the diagnosis provides no information about severity, and if more complete information on the patient were available, designations other than D or E could be made. But categories D and E differ in that category E diagnoses will usually permit discretion on whether and how to treat the patient.

The results of grouping the 1,907 hospitalizations for our sample of 16,000 Medicaid eligibles are shown in table 15–5. On the basis of physician discretion regarding hospitalization, clearly the OPDs and private physi-

Table 15–5
Distribution of Hospital Diagnoses by Degree of Discretion, Source of Care, and Eligibility Status, California, 1976–1978

Diagnosis Group	Eligibility Status	Predominant Source of Care		(Private Office Less OPD) (Percent)
		Private Office (Percent)	OPD (Percent)	
A, B. Definite hospitaliza-	AFDC female	34.4	56.4	−22.0
tion; no choice of timing	Disabled	19.0	23.7	−4.7
C. Definite hospitalization;	AFDC female	11.5	3.8	7.7
quality-of-life choice;	Disabled	8.0	4.3	3.7
generally nonurgent				
D. Don't know; not enough	AFDC female	19.9	12.7	7.2
information	Disabled	28.5	26.8	1.7
E. Treatment modality and	AFDC female	25.8	23.8	2.0
hospitalization open to	Disabled	34.2	29.5	4.7
choice and judgment				
F. Usually not hospitalized	AFDC female	8.1	3.3	4.8
	Disabled	10.3	15.8	−5.5
Total	AFDC female	100.0	100.0	0
	Disabled	100.0	100.0	

cians' offices had a different patient mix. For example, for AFDC females who were hospitalized and whose predominant source of care was an OPD, over half the hospitalization diagnoses (56.4 percent) were in categories A and B (that is, urgent with no discretion). For the disabled, the differences in categories A and B across source of care were similar although not as dramatic, with 24 and 19 percent for OPD and private practice, respectively.

The pattern is reversed for discretionary quality-of-life hospitalization (category C): Hospitalized patients (in both Medicaid groups) from private offices have greater proportions in this category than do the patients from OPDs. Category E, which involves discretion and choice of treatment modality, was also more frequently observed among patients from private offices than patients from OPDs, although the differences were small. The unknown category (D) was also more weighted toward the private office.

An overview of these frequencies suggests that in terms of physician discretion regarding hospitalization, it appears that the patients from OPDs are more likely to have diagnoses in the less discretionary categories (A and B). In other words, a greater proportion of the hospitalized patients from OPDs are hospitalized for conditions that have little or no physician discretion, and more patients from private offices are hospitalized for conditions that involve physician discretion or choice (C).

The preceding discussion has focused on the hospital-discharge diagnosis. In terms of discretionary care, it could be argued that some settings of care may treat discretionary cases on an outpatient basis—which would mean that such care would not appear as an inpatient record. Therefore, we also constructed an index of selected surgical procedures and determined whether they were done on an inpatient or outpatient basis. Table 15–6 shows the distributions of these categories of surgical procedures by PSC. These data confirm the hypothesis that compared to private-practice patients, patients whose predominant source of care was an OPD received dramatically less discretionary surgery. Both the AFDC females and the disabled patients from private offices receive three and a half to four and a half times more discretionary surgery than do the OPD patients. While the patients from OPDs tended to receive a smaller proportion of their discretionary surgery on an inpatient basis compared to the patients from private offices, the differences were not enough to contradict the previous result regarding classification of the inpatient diagnoses. In sum, the selected discretionary surgical procedures clearly show that patients from OPDs received less discretionary surgical care than did the patients from private offices.

Returning to the hospital diagnoses of categories A and B (no discretion), what were the diagnoses that were so significant for the OPD, and how does this finding affect our basic focus on the cost of medical care across different settings? Not surprisingly, normal delivery is the most frequent

Table 15-6
Mean Selected "Discretionary" Surgical Procedures for Medicaid Eligibles, by Predominant Source of Care and Eligibility Status, California, 1976-1978

Measure	Eligibility Status[b]	Predominant Source of Care[a]		Total[c]
		Private Office	OPD	
Total dollars paid	Female AFDC	1.48	0.35	0.97
	Disabled	2.94	0.65	1.69
Inpatient dollars as a percent of total	Female AFDC	44.15	38.58	43.98
	Disabled	53.04	3.68	50.30
Total RVUs	Female AFDC	3.00	0.86	1.96
	Disabled	7.14	0.04	4.02
Inpatient RVUs as a percent of total	Female AFDC	51.84	50.72	51.90
	Disabled	57.91	3.57	55.92
Total visits	Female AFDC	0.04	0.02	0.03
	Disabled	0.12	0.03	0.07
Inpatient visits as a percent of total	Female AFDC	21.63	12.31	19.85
	Disabled	7.99	5.26	8.14

Note: *Discretionary surgical procedures* are eleven procedures that generally require the discretion of the physician. Examples include arthrocentesis and cataract extraction.

[a]*Predominant source of care* is defined as the setting where the maximum number of ambulatory visits occurred.

[b]Based on a sample of 8,622 female AFDC eligibles not eligible for prepaid care and eligible for at least six continuous months. Those aged seven to fourteen years old and those aged sixty-five or older are excluded. Los Angeles and drug claims are excluded. Data are weighted to correct for age cohort and geographic stratification. The disabled statistics are based on a sample of 8,151 disabled eligibles. Those sixty-five or older are excluded. Los Angeles County and drug claims are excluded.

[c]Includes all sources of care, not just the two categories shown here.

diagnosis in categories A and B for AFDC females, and for some reason OPDs have a larger proportion of the total deliveries. (It is a separate issue as to why OPDs have a greater proportion of pregnancies than do private offices. Anecdotal accounts indicate that the fee schedule is such that private obstetricians in California are less willing to treat pregnant Medicaid women.) In fact, the hospitalization rate for females treated in an OPD drops from 20 percent with deliveries to 10 percent without deliveries.

Because of the age distribution of the disabled, pregnancies are not generally an issue, and there are no obvious conditions that explain the greater proportion of the disabled hospitalizations in categories A and B for OPDs than for private-office patients. It should be recalled that the difference in categories A and B for the disabled between OPDs and private offices while substantial was small compared to AFDC women—24 versus 19 percent (see table 15-5).

A more complete comparison of the effect of removing pregnancies for the AFDC population is shown in table 15–7. With pregnancies removed, we observe that average total cost per beneficiary for six months for patients treated in an OPD was lower ($264) than the cost for patients treated in private offices ($307). This change in the relative rankings between OPDs and private offices was a consequence of the lowered hospitalizations, which actually increased the average inpatient costs for the private-practice patients slightly. For OPD patients, however, the average inpatient costs decreased 60 percent, from $297 to $120.

An overview of the data in table 15–7 shows a much less dramatic story in hospitalization rates and total costs across these settings of ambulatory care for the AFDC population. Without pregnancies, the differences are small. It is not possible to definitively state whether the patients choosing these settings are different, other than the obvious case of pregnant women who are more likely to have an OPD as a source of care than a private physician's office. The clearly observed, nonrandom pattern for pregnancies is some indication of "self-selection" by patients, but whether this extends to other conditions or along severity lines within given conditions, we cannot say conclusively. For example, the category D of hospital diagnosis (not enough information) could be reasonably similar in the aggregate, yet within this category there could be systematic differences so that one or the other setting of care would receive more severe cases requiring more hospitalizations. We cannot refute or support such a hypothesis.

Let us now return to the other four potential explanations (table 15–4) for the higher hospitalization rates for patients using an outpatient department as their PSC. What have these data and analyses shown? First, it would

Table 15–7
Comparison of Cost per Eligible and Percent Hospitalized for All AFDC Recipients and with Deliveries Excluded

Eligibility Status	Cost Parameter	Predominant Source of Care[a]					
		Private Physician's Office		Hospital OPD		Total[b]	
Female AFDC	Percent hospitalized	11	(9)	20	(10)	9	(8)
	Inpatient costs	$130	($110)	$297	($120)	$121	($111)
	Percent of total	44	(46)	62	(45)	48	(47)
	Total costs	$296	($307)	$477	($264)	$251	($234)

Note: Data in parentheses are for the same basic samples of eligibles except that women with a delivery in the six months of observation have been removed.

[a]Defined to be the mode (most frequent) of the setting where patients received their ambulatory physician visits.

[b]Includes all eligibles across all the sources of care and not just the two shown here.

appear that there is some truth to the first potential hypothesis, that is, the mix of patients in the two settings is different. Specifically, the frequency of category A and B hospitalization diagnoses (no discretion) are such that much of the difference in hospitalization rates can be explained by case-mix differences. This is true for both the disabled and the AFDC female eligibles, with pregnancies being of particular importance for the latter. We do not think these results are conclusive, but clearly there are differences across PSC of private practice and OPD such that there is support for this basic hypothesis.

This analysis has not shed much light on the second and third potential explanations given earlier in the chapter, that is, not much can be said on the potential differences in physicians practicing in OPDs or in differences in the interaction of patients and physicians in the OPD. As for the fourth explanation regarding possible venal behavior of physicians practicing in OPDs, while these results are not conclusive, the data on discretionary hospital diagnoses (category C in table 15–4) and on selected discretionary surgical procedures (table 15–6) do not support the fill-the-bed hypothesis. If physicians were going to help keep the hospital full for nonmedical reasons, it would seem that a likely starting point would be discretionary surgery.

Another item that tends to militate against hypothesis 4 is the absence of a dramatically higher hospitalization rate for patients with a PSC of the emergency room compared to patients from private-practice sources of care.

Case-Mix Differences and a Comparison with the Lion-Altman Results

A fundamental finding of the Lion-Altman research is that the case mixes of patients seen in OPDs and patients seen in private practices are substantially similar in terms of case complexity; and if there are differences, they are small with perhaps OPD patients' being "15 percent more complex."[9] How should the results of our analysis be compared with those of Lion and Altman?

First of all, it should be noted that there were substantial differences in the methodology and populations studied. Lion and Altman analyzed patient-physician contacts from a national sample of primary-care physicians. They specifically excluded all visits to an emergency room and all visits to obstetricians and gynecologists. Our sample, by contrast, was restricted to two subsets of the California Medicaid population. In addition, our sample focused on a six-month patient history and considered all sources of care, including emergency-room visits and visits to obstetricians and gynecologists. Consequently, the comparisons between Lion and Altman and our results have some definite limits. However, we believe that there are enough similarities in the populations studied and interest in the topic to list some likely areas of agreement and differences between the two studies.

First, the areas of agreement: Excluding pregnant women and their greater proclivity to use an OPD rather than a private physician's office, it would appear that the *magnitude* of the likely differences in "patient complexity" between the two settings is not extraordinary. Our conclusions are generally based on the intensity of physician visits in the two settings and on the likelihood of hospitalization. We are not as confident of the precise magnitude of the differences as are Lion and Altman, but the data of this project would not be consistent with reimbursements for OPDs two or three times as great as private physicians receive based on case complexity. While differences of this magnitude may seem absurd to some, such differences are not unlikely in some Medicaid programs. For example, New York State currently has a $60 ceiling on the reimbursement of physician visits in an OPD.[10]

In the areas of disagreement between our results and Lion and Altman: The significant use of the OPD for obstetrical and gynecological care suggests that there are case-mix differences between OPDs and private practices. Lion and Altman, of course, have excluded such visits from their analysis, but it would seem that this is a critical exclusion with significant implications. The differences in categories A and B hospitalizations (no discretion), which include deliveries but other conditions as well, suggests that the case-mix differences extend beyond Ob-Gyn, especially when one considers the disabled who are not likely users of Ob-Gyn services. These differences in case mix may or may not contradict Lion and Altman's results about case complexity per se, but these differences are not consistent with the notion that OPDs and private practices treat the same mix of patients. We certainly know these differences in case mix lead to dramatic differences in the use of inpatient care. We are uncertain of their precise impact on the cost of ambulatory care.

Implications and Conclusions

Basically, states follow one of two methods for reimbursing providers of medical services. The first is cost reimbursement whereby providers receive "the cost" of care, which is usually an accounting estimate of average costs per day or per service. This method, which has traditionally been used to reimburse short-term hospitals for inpatient care, has come under increasing criticism because of the incentive for providers to always provide both more care and more expensive care. Many states reimburse outpatient visits to OPDs and emergency rooms on this basis.

The other method of reimbursement for medical services is a charge system whereby a provider receives a predetermined, fixed amount for a given service. This method is frequently used to reimburse physicians under a variant called a fee schedule, that is, a set of fixed, predetermined prices for a given set of services.

During the period of this study, California Medicaid reimbursed practically all providers of physician services on a charge system. While California was similar to most states in reimbursing for physician visits provided in a private office on a charge basis, it was somewhat atypical in also paying for physician visits in an OPD on a charge basis. Only a distinct minority of states use a fee schedule for OPD services, with half of the states' reimbursing for OPD services on a cost basis.[11] In any case, it is most likely that this OPD-payment method has strong implications for how providers respond in their treatment of Medicaid patients, and the results just presented are probably dependent on this OPD-reimbursement method. In other words, *the costs and patterns of care, as reported here, are in part a consequence of the payment method*, and generalizing from these results needs to take account of the differences that may exist in payment methods among states.

It appears then that one of the significant findings of this study is that OPDs per se do not need to be extraordinarily costly places for ambulatory care. More precisely, the analysis presented suggests that differences between private practices and OPDs in total program costs per patient month, in a state that uses charge reimbursement for both the OPD and private practice, need not be that dramatically different.[12] More refined analyses as part of this or future projects may show differences in costs that may offer opportunities for cost savings through appropriate restructuring of incentives. However, it seems clear from these data that the magnitude of the savings will be substantially less than that which common folklore suggests.

Determining the charge the state should pay for a service is not easy. Setting the charge too low is likely to decrease access or quality since providers will be less willing to treat patients at that price. Setting the price too high will cost the program more than the social value of the services provided.[13] Ultimately it is a political and social judgment that must be made about where and what services the public wants to purchase for the Medicaid population.[14]

Many positive things can be said about a charge-based system such as that used by California for reimbursing hospital OPD. Such a system gives the hospital an incentive to minimize costs, although technically this is true only if the hospital maximizes profits, which may or may not be true for nonprofit hospitals. In addition, if similar services are reimbursed at the same rate regardless of where received (for example, private office or OPD), then providers and patients have incentives to choose among alternatives based on medical, ethical, and other values; that is, the fiscal incentives are not needlessly distorting the choice structure.

While the preceding analysis has focused on the issue of total program costs per patient month, it might be repeated that the cost of ambulatory care is only a minor part of the total costs. If ambulatory costs are controlled via a charge-reimbursement system, it is the potential abuse of the admitting power to the hospital that should be of public concern. The results discussed here show that within reasonable bounds of precision and our currently available data, it does not appear that the admission power of OPDs has been seriously abused if private-practice physicians are used as a standard of comparison.

Notes

1. D.N. Muse and D. Sawyer, *The Medicaid and Medicare Data Book, 1981*, U.S. Department of Health and Human Services (Washington, D.C.: Health Care Financing Administration, 1982), p. 25.

2. *Economic Report of the President, 1982* (Washington, D.C.: Government Printing Office, 1982), table B-53.

3. Muse and Sawyer, *Medicaid and Medicare Data Book*, p. 34. For Medicare expenditures, the rate of uninsured in hospital outpatient services was even greater at 27 percent per year, compounded.

4. Joanna Lion and Stuart Altman, "Case Mix Differences Between Hospital Outpatient Departments and Private Practice," *Health Care Financing Review*, vol. 4, no. 1, Sept. 1982.

5. Also see Philip J. Held and Katherine Swartz, "Physician Fees and the Cost of Medicaid," The Urban Institute, Washington, D.C., 1983, forthcoming. Also see Carol Hamcke, "Where Medicaid Patients Receive Their Ambulatory Care," The Urban Institute, Washington, D.C., 1983, forthcoming.

6. *Health, United States, 1978*, Public Health Service, Department of Health, Education and Welfare Publication No. (HRA) 78–1272, p. 268.

7. Held and Swartz, 1983.

8. Lion and Altman, 1982.

9. Ibid.

10. Personal communication, New York State Department of Social Services.

11. Muse and Sawyer, op. cit., pp. 116–118. California had a charge-based system for reimbursing physician visits in an OPD, with some discounting of the fees compared to what physicians in private offices receive. In the first year of this study, the discount was 40 percent, but it was reduced to 20 percent in the latter two years (1977–1978).

12. Personal communication, California Department of Health Services. California hospitals were not particularly happy about the level of

reimbursement they were receiving from Medicaid for OPD services. They argued that the charge should be linked to costs and that their costs exceeded what the state was willing to pay. Apparently, a substantial legal suit brought by the California Hospital Association argued that paying charges independent of costs was an inappropriate basis for the state to use in reimbursing hospital OPDs. The case was decided in favor of the state.

13. We are ignoring any effects of the setting of ambulatory services on the use of inpatient care. See Held and Swartz, "Physician Fees."

14. For more details on the topic of what charges should be, see Philip J. Held and Mark V. Pauly, *Competition and Efficiency in the End Stage Renal Disease Programs* (Washington, D.C.: The Urban Institute, 1982).

Name Index

Subject Index

Access, appointment times, 29, 32, 168; inner city residents, 3–4, 8–9, 13, 27, 73–74, 89, 95, 138, 177; racial differences in, 14–15; rural residents, 13, 95; related to income, 14; travel time, 18–19, 31–32, 142

Alcoholism, 32, 113, 166–167

Ambulatory visit groups (AVGs), 163–164

American Hospital Association, 87, 95–96, 162, 181–182; Commission on Public General Hospitals, 137

American Medical Association, 137, 161, 171

Ancillary services, as part of visit, 80, 118, 120, 132, 180; equipment used in, 133; insurance for, 54, 58; repetition of tests, 29, 33; revenue from, 5, 93, 98–99, 117–118

Angiography, digital subtraction, 133

Bad debts, 71, 73, 115

Beth Israel Ambulatory Care Center (BIAC), description of, 111–114; utilization of, 165, 171

Beth Israel Hospital, 5–6, 111, 118

Billing arrangements, hospital OPDs, 83–84

Black Caucus, U.S. Congress, 34

Blacks, prevalence of illness for, 28; third party payer coverage for, 14; use of OPDs 27, 30

Blood glucose monitoring devices, 125–128

Blue Cross/Blue Shield, 1, 3, 53–62; contractural discount, 150; coverage of OPD care, 54–55, 116–118; HMOs, 148

Boston City Hospital (BCH), 165

Brookings Institution, 140

California Health Facilities Commission (CHFC), 181–182, 187, 193

California Hospital Association, 213

Capitation, HMOs, 148, 150; primary care, 23, 74

Cardiac-monitoring devices, 126, 128

Case management, 74, 147

Case mix, measurement of, 48–49; medical, 2, 7–8, 161, 166–167, 175–176, 179–180; social, 2, 7–8, 161–162, 169–177, 180

Center for Health Administration Studies (CHAS), University of Chicago, 140–141

Charges, OPD compared with free-standing clinics, 59

Co-insurance, applied to Medicaid, 41; applied to Medicare, 39

Columbia University, College of Physicians and Surgeons, 30

Community Development Block Grants, 144

Community Health Centers, 13, 20–23, 31–32, 70, 138; admitting privileges for physicians, 33, 145

Community Hospital Program (CHP), 91–92, 97, 107–108; fiscal viability of, 102–103; organizational structure of OPDs, 105–107

Conservation of Human Resources (CHR), Columbia University, 140–142

Continuity of care, 29, 92, 202–203; computerized records, 32–33, 92, 114

Corporate structure, relationship between hospital and OPD, 83–84, 130

Cost, differences between sites, 7, 21; marginal of providing OPD visit, 87–88; per visit community health centers, 21; per visit OPDs, 6, 8, 59, 66, 100–101, 183–187; per visit physician groups, 183–185, 190–191

Cost allocation, 40, 118, 180; for OPDs, 85

Cost limits, hospital (Section 223), 131

Cost shifting, among payers, 9; from inpatient to OPD, 5, 48, 68, 130

216

Conference Participants

Frederick Ackroyd, M.D.
Surgical Services
Mount Sinai Medical Center
Miami Beach, Florida

Stuart H. Altman, Ph.D.
Dean, Heller Graduate School
Brandeis University
Waltham, Massachusetts

Richard Berman, M.P.A.
Commissioner, New York State
    Division of Housing and
    Community Renewal
New York, New York

Irwin Birnbaum, J.D.
Vice-President for Finance
Montefiore Hospital and Medical
    Center
Bronx, New York

Robert Blendon, Sc.D.
Vice-President, Planning and
    Development
Robert Wood Johnson Foundation
Princeton, New Jersey

Jerome F. Brazda
Executive Editor
McGraw-Hill's *Washington Health
    Letters*
Washington, D.C.

Charles Brecher, Ph.D.
Associate Professor
Graduate School of Public
    Administration
New York University
New York, New York

Bonnie Brickett, M.P.H.
Program Analyst
Office of the Assistant Secretary
    for Planning and Evaluation
Department of Health and Human
    Services
Washington, D.C.

Linda A. Burns, M.H.A.
Director, Division of Ambulatory
    Care
American Hospital Association
Chicago, Illinois

Gary A. Christopherson, M.S.
Assistant Director
Municipal Health Services Program
Johns Hopkins University
Baltimore, Maryland

Robert M. Crane, M.B.A.
Director, Office of Health Systems
    Management
New York State Department of
    Health
Albany, New York

Karen Davis, Ph.D.
Department of Health Care
    Organization
School of Public Health
Johns Hopkins University
Baltimore, Maryland

Thomas Delbanco, M.D.
Medical Director
Beth Israel Ambulatory Care
Boston, Massachusetts

James E. DeLozier, M.S.
Chief, Ambulatory Care Statistics
   Branch
Division of Health Care Statistics
National Center for Health Statistics
Hyattsville, Maryland

David Dolins, M.P.H.
Executive Vice-President and
   Director
Beth Israel Hospital
Boston, Massachusetts

Sandra L. Fenwick, M.P.H.
Associate Director
Beth Israel Hospital
Boston, Massachusetts

Richard Foster, Ph.D.
Assistant Professor
Center for Health Administration
   Studies
Graduate School of Business
University of Chicago
Chicago, Illinois

Clifton Gaus, Sc.D.
Director, Center for Health Policy
   Studies
Georgetown University
Washington, D.C.

Paul Gertman, M.D.
Director of Health Care Research
University Hospital
Boston, Massachusetts

Marsha Gold, Sc.D.
Director, Policy Analysis and
   Program Evaluation
Maryland Department of Health
   and Mental Hygiene
Baltimore, Maryland

Donald Goldstone, M.D.
Acting Director
National Center for Health Services
   Research
Hyattsville, Maryland

Fay Hannon, M.B.A., C.P.A.
Cambridge, Massachusetts

Philip J. Held, Ph.D.
The Urban Institute
Washington, D.C.

Mary G. Henderson, M.M.H.S.
Research Analyst
Heller School
Brandeis University
Waltham, Massachusetts

Neil Hollander, M.S.
Executive Director
Blue Cross & Blue Shield
   Association
Chicago, Illinois

John Iglehart,
Editor
Health Affairs
Potomac, Maryland

Richard M. Knapp, Ph.D.
Director, Department of Teaching
   Hospitals
American Association of Medical
   Colleges
Washington, D.C.

Jackson W. Knowlton, M.P.A.
Administrative Director
Council on Health Care Financing
Albany, New York

Mary Alice Krill, Ph.D.
Center for Research in Ambulatory
   Health Care Administration
Medical Group Management
   Association
Denver, Colorado

Richard Laird, M.H.A.
Director of Ambulatory Services
University Hospitals of Cleveland
Cleveland, Ohio

Joanna Lion, Ph.D.
Senior Research Associate and
   Ambulatory Care Study Director
Heller Graduate School
Brandeis University
Waltham, Massachusetts

Lorna McBarnette, M.S., M.P.H.
Vice-President, Clinical and
   Ambulatory Services
Saint Peter's Hospital
Albany, New York

Gregory E. McKinney, M.H.A.
Program Management Policy Officer
Georgia Department of Medical
   Assistance
Altanta, Georgia

Alan J. Malbon
Director, Research and
   Development
Mackie-Decker Associates
Newton Highlands, Massachusetts

Henry Miller, Ph.D.
President, Center for Health Policy
   Studies, Inc.
Columbia, Maryland

Robert A. Musacchio, Ph.D.
Research Economist
Department of Medical Practice
   Economics
Center for Health Policy Research
American Medical Association
Chicago, Illinois

Herluf C. Olsen, M.H.A.
Group Vice-President
American Hospital Association
Chicago, Illinois

Louis A. Orsini
Vice-President, Health Insurance
   Association of America
New York, New York

David R. Ott
Vice-President, United Hospital
   Fund of New York
New York, New York

Stanley B. Peck
Health Insurance Association of
   America
New York, New York

Robert J. Peoples, M.A.
Executive Vice-President and Chief
   Operating Officer
Samaritan Health Center
Detroit, Michigan

Nancy Alfored Persily, M.P.H.
Director of Planning
Mount Sinai Medical Center
Miami, Florida

Charles Rangel (R.-N.Y.)
Chairman, Subcommittee on
 Oversight and Investigations
Committee on Ways and Means
U.S. House of Representatives
Washington, D.C.

Diane Rowland, M.P.H.
Department of Health Care
 Organization
School of Public Health
Johns Hopkins University
Baltimore, Maryland

Edward Salsberg, M.P.A.
Director, Primary Care and Health
 Professions Coordination Unit
New York State Department of
 Health
Albany, New York

Lyda B. Sanford, M.L.A.
Chief, Division of Program
 Development and Analysis
Medical Assistance Administration
Department of Health and Mental
 Hygiene
Baltimore, Maryland

George J. Schieber, Ph.D.
Director, Office of Policy Analysis
Health Care Financing
 Administration
Washington, D.C.

Carl J. Schramm, Ph.D.
Health Services Administration
School of Public Health
Johns Hopkins University
Baltimore, Maryland

Edward Shapiro
President, Mount Sinai Medical
 Center Foundation
Miami Beach, Florida

Stuart Shapiro, M.D.
Commissioner of Health
City of Philadelphia
Department of Public Health
Philadelphia, Pennsylvania

Mary Stuart, M.C.P.
Assistant to the Assistant Secretary
 for Medical Care Programs
Department of Health and Mental
 Hygiene
Baltimore, Maryland

Charles M. Taylor, M.P.A.
Administrative Director
Urban Health Network Program
University of Wisconsin, Madison
Madison, Wisconsin

Howard R. Veit, M.H.A.
Executive Director
The Philadelphia Health Plan
Philadelphia, Pennsylvania

James Vertrees, Ph.D.
Project Officer, Health Care
 Financing Administration
Washington, D.C.

Stanley S. Wallack, Ph.D.
Director, University Health Policy
 Consortium
Heller School
Brandeis University
Waltham, Massachusetts

Henry Waxman (D.-Calif.)
Chairman, Subcommittee on Health
 and the Environment
Committee on Interstate and
 Foreign Commerce
U.S.House of Representatives
Washington, D.C.

Thomas M. Wickizer, M.P.H.
Research Associate and Project
  Director
Community Hospital Program
  Evaluation
Department of Health Services
School of Public Health and
  Community Medicine
University of Washington
Seattle, Washington

Judith LaVor Williams, Ph.D.
Research Associate
Heller School
Brandeis University
Waltham, Massachusetts

Donald A. Young, M.D.
Acting Deputy Director
Bureau of Program Policy
Health Care Financing
  Administration
Baltimore, Maryland

Quentin Young, M.D.
Hyde Park Associates in Medicine
Chicago, Illinois

Michael Ziegler, J.D.
Epstein, Becker
Borsodoy, Greene
New York, New York

About the Contributors

Ronald M. Andersen, Ph.D., is the director of the Center for Health Administration Studies and the Graduate Program in Hospital Administration at the University of Chicago, where he is also a professor.

Beverly Birns, Ph.D., is a professor in the Social Science Interdisciplinary Program, Psychology, and the Department of Psychiatry, at the State University of New York at Stony Brook. As a Congressional Science Fellow, she worked as a special assistant to Congressman Charles B. Rangel.

Charles Brecher, Ph.D., is an associate professor at the New York University Graduate School of Public Administration and is codirector of the Setting Municipal Priorities project in New York City.

Linda A. Burns, M.H.A., is the director of the Division of Ambulatory Care at the American Hospital Association.

Robert M. Crane, M.H.A., is the director of the New York State Office for Health Systems Management. He has also served on the staff of the Subcommittee of Health and the Environment, U.S. House of Representatives.

Edith M. Davis is a senior research associate at the Conservation of Human Resources, Columbia University, and the project director of Municipal Health Services Program Evaluation.

Karen Davis, Ph.D., is a professor in the School of Hygiene and Public Health and the Department of Political Economy of The Johns Hopkins University. She previously served as Administrator of the Public Health Service Health Resources Administration and as Deputy Assistant Secretary for Planning and Evaluation/Health at the Department of Health and Human Services.

Thomas L. Delbanco, M.D., is the director of the Division of General Medicine and Primary Care, Beth Israel Hospital, and an associate professor of medicine at Harvard Medical School.

David Ehrenfried is a consultant on the development of cost-containment programs with the Health Care Services Department of the Blue Cross and Blue Shield Association, Chicago.

Gretchen Voorhis Fleming, Ph.D., is a senior research associate at the Center for Health Administration Studies, University of Chicago.

Fay L. Hannon, M.B.A., C.P.A., is a consultant to the Heller School, Brandeis University, in hospital cost accounting.

Philip J. Held, Ph.D., is a senior research associate at The Urban Institute, Washington, D.C.

Mary G. Henderson, M.M.H.S., is a research associate at the Heller School, Brandeis University.

Neil Hollander, M.S., is the executive director of the Health Care Services Department, Blue Cross and Blue Shield Association, Chicago.

Harvey J. Makadon, M.D., is the medical director of Emergency and General Medical Outpatient Services, Beth Israel Hospital. He is also an instructor in medicine at Harvard Medical School.

Miriam Ostow is a senior research associate at the Conservation of Human Resources, Columbia University.

Charles B. Rangel is a member of the U.S. House of Representatives from New York. He is the chairman of the Ways and Means Subcommittee on Oversight and Investigation and is a member of the Select Committee on Narcotics Abuse and Control and the Democratic Steering and Policy Committee.

Edward S. Salsberg, M.P.A., is the director of the Primary Care and Health Professions Coordination Unit, Division of Program and Policy Development and Evaluation, at the New York State Department of Health.

George J. Schieber, Ph.D., is the director of the Office of Policy Analysis, Health Care Financing Administration, at the Department of Health and Human Services.

Stephen M. Shortell, Ph.D., is the A.C. Buehler Distinguished Professor of Hospital and Health Services Management and a professor of organization behavior at the J. L. Kellogg Graduate School of Management, Northwestern University, Evanston.

Katherine Swartz, Ph.D., is a research associate at The Urban Institute, Washington, D.C.

Howard R. Veit, M.H.A., is the executive director of the Philadelphia Health Plan and an executive with Hancock Dikewood Associates, which manages the plan. Previously he headed the federal health-maintenance-organization (HMO) program.

Thomas M. Wickizer, M.P.H., is the project director of the Community Hospital Program Evaluation, Department of Health Services, School of Public Health and Community Medicine, University of Washington, Seattle.

Michele S. Winsten, M.S., is assistant director at Beth Israel Hospital, and lecturer at the Harvard School of Public Health.

Donald A. Young, M.D., is the acting deputy director of the Bureau of Program Policy, Health Care Financing Administration, Department of Health and Human Services.

About the Editors

Stuart H. Altman received the Ph.D. from the University of California at Los Angeles and is currently the dean of the Florence Heller Graduate School for Advanced Studies in Social Welfare, Brandeis University. Dr. Altman serves as the chairman of the Board of Governors of the University Health Policy Consortium. From 1971 to 1976, he was the deputy assistant secretary for planning and evaluation at the Department of Health, Education and Welfare and the deputy director for health of the Cost-of-Living Council.

Joanna Lion received the Ph.D. from the University of Chicago and is now a senior research associate at the Heller School. She is the study director for a four-year project, funded by the Robert Wood Johnson Foundation and the Department of Health and Human Services, that will study the costs of ambulatory care. Her health-care background includes ten years as a research director for two state-hospital associations.

Judith LaVor Williams received the Ph.D. from Brandeis University and is a research associate at the Heller School. She has been working on the ambulatory-care project looking at socioeconomic case mix. Before coming to the Heller School, Dr. Williams was responsible for long-term-care demonstrations and policy analysis at the Health Care Financing Administration, Department of Health and Human Services.